M000221858

Too Tired to Cook

The Guide to Choosing Foods that Will Boost Your Energy and Enhance Your Immune System

Mary L. Higgins, B.S., M.Ed

This book is designed to provide accurate and authoritative information on Nutrition. It should be used in consultation with your health care provider. For a specific health problem, please consult your physician. While every attempt has been made to provide accurate nutrition information as of the date of publication, the author cannot be held responsible for any errors or omissions. The author disclaims any liability for any medical outcomes that may occur as a result of following the information in this book. This book is not intended to replace a personal consultation with a health professional who is familiar with your medical history.

10 9 8 7 6 5 4 3 2 1

Interior formatting and cover design: Rachael Ritchey, RR Publishing

Melting woman graphic design: Michael Swerkle

With love to my
Dear Mother and Father
who made writing this book possible

TABLE OF CONTENTS

INTRODUCTION

Pick up the kids; drop the kids off at soccer practice; wait in line at the post office; Drive to the ATM; take the kids back home, cook dinner. DINNER? There's no time, and you are barely able to stand up from exhaustion.

This book is for you.

You work all day listening to other's complaints, enduring that bumper-to-bumper traffic on the long commute home. You just want to put your feet up, open some wine, and rest. Entering the kitchen, you suddenly realize, you forgot to defrost the chicken. Now what?

This book is for you, too.

Do you suffer from an illness that exhausts you? Fatigue plays a supporting role in many medical conditions, so many of them chronic and unrelenting. It takes effort to walk into the kitchen, let alone, spend time in front of the stove cooking an entire meal. Do you find it a challenge to prepare a meal when you used all your energy just to get through the day? Did you survive Covid19, yet the lingering effects of the virus have left you dizzy and tired, no longer with the stamina you once had?

If so, you will positively love this book!

PREFACE

Billions of dollars in U.S. productivity are lost due to both chronic and acute illness preventing people from being able to work, and this was before Covid19 ever hit our shores. In its first 6 months, the virus killed 200,000 Americans. Thousands more were left with damage to several vital organs, including the heart muscle making the simplest errands become a challenge. There is hope. That's why you picked up this book. While there are no medicines that can magically supply us energy and bring us back to where we were before our illness hit, there are foods that can help. Did you know the foods we eat can either ENERGIZE us or cause a mid-day *crash?* You want to feel healthy and energetic, right? Isn't that why you picked up this book?

Not everyone is destined to "suffer" the conditions that creep in after our 30's and beyond that many of us contend with, although we start to age the day we are born and begin to feel it in our mid-twenties (when staying up to 2 a.m every night is no longer possible). Other conditions, such as high blood pressure, high cholesterol, irritable bowel, or stiff and painful joints, just to name a few, are NOT inevitable. Do you know you can play a pivotal role in preventing yourself from suffering with these? Even if your family tree is genetically stacked against you; you can alter your destiny. For example, Arthritis, which can be so debilitating, from both pain and fatigue, may be avoided with the inclusion of specific nutrients in our diets. Food can be powerful medicine! Some nutrients have the ability to heal our bodies of inflammation as well as pain even after being diagnosed with an illness. And the best part is, you don't need to spend hundreds of dollars on expensive supplements. Foods with their all-inclusive package of nutrients, can be a powerful ally in our efforts to stay healthy!

Research now confirms many diseases with "fatigue" as a central feature involve INFLAMMATION, a filthy word, at its base. Diseases including arthritis, heart disease, asthma, colitis to name just few. Although these disparate illnesses may not seem to have much in common, since they involve different parts of the body, they share one thing, INFLAMMATION. Inflammation can be as simple and short-lived as a headache or encompass multiple body systems as in autoimmune illnesses. Our immune system sends chemical messengers to places in the body where injury occurs, to ramp up the production of white blood cells to heal the injured, i.e., inflamed area. In the case of a disease, the injury starts at the cellular level. You've probably heard of two pain messengers mentioned during TV ads for pain relievers; *prostaglandins* and *leukotrienes.* These are responsible for any kind of pain, including menstrual cramps we women know can be very debilitating.

At a cellular level, these pain-producing chemicals, are created in abnormal amounts and go on to irritate tissue, causing swelling, pain, and fatigue. By enjoying nutrient-rich foods and skillfully avoiding others, we can actually prevent these damaging chemical messengers from flooding our bodies. Along with inflammation, substances called *free radicals* are created every day with the potential to cause further damage to every tissue in the body, especially our DNA, the genetic material that tells our cells what actions to take. By eating foods rich in protective factors called *anti-oxidants*, we may limit the amount of free radicals.

You may be surprised to learn that free radicals are everywhere: in car exhaust, air fresheners, radon, plastics, radiation, even STRESS can cause these substances to build up in our bodies. Did you know activities that are good for us, such as exercise, if done to excess, may promote the production of free radicals inside our bodies?

Just like a car that receives high octane fuel, a body receiving the right nutrients runs longer and more efficiently, accumulating fewer free radicals. How many of you are unhappy with the shape of your body or with your weight? How many diets have you endured to get rid of that "muffin top" or "love handles" just to fit into your favorite pair of pants? You can rid of yourself of that unwanted fat and gain the upper hand over your metabolism just by giving your body the nutrients that it really needs, and you may not even need to restrict your calories!

One of the leading causes of death in this country, coming in at #2, is Cancer. Unknown to many people, every human body, even a healthy one, contains a certain number of cancerous cells, that hang around inside us. Still, a healthy immune system is capable of disarming the invading cancer cells so that their population doesn't grow out of control, causing tumors. Those of us with chronic illness are under siege from free radicals, so we need to be extra diligent in providing anti-oxidant rich foods to flood every cell in our bodies with the nutrients they deserve. Let's banish the bad guys—those free radicals—from the premises.

This book will show you ways to strengthen your immune system, decrease pain and fatigue, and rid your body of accumulated free radicals and oxidative stress. What is oxidative stress? It is a sort of "wear and tear" that arises simply from aging, which first occurs inside our cells. Those of us us with chronic illness experience more "wear and tear" and the medications we take to control our symptoms, because they need to be processed by our liver, increase the amount of work this organ needs to do to break down the toxic load. In the process of doing that, we can become even sicker, if our metabolic pathways have damage.

ACKNOWLEDGMENTS

For their help in the making of *Too Tired to Cook*, I would like to thank the following people: Michael Swerkle for his graphic design. A grateful thank you to Teddy Kalfopoulos, Margie Melaragni and Kendall Dudley for their contributions to the initial manuscript; Virginia Covino and Jerry Fox, wonderful friends and readers who kept me motivated to continue writing, my mother for help with the editing, and my incredible formatter and cover designer, Rachael Ritchey. I want to thank Julia Fox Garrison, author of *Don't Leave Me This Way!* I met this extraordinary woman at the Newburyport Literary Festival and she encouraged me to pursue my book idea. My acknowledgements would not be complete without a special thank you to Chandler Bolt for his inspiration, encouragement and the knowledge to bring the ball over the goal post.

Too Tired to Cook

CHAPTER 1

According to the Centers for Disease Control website, many chronic illnesses feature fatigue as one component or even the primary one. Maybe you got diagnosed with multiple sclerosis, an autoimmune condition, cardiovascular disease, cancer, or a neuromuscular disease, maybe even Chronic Fatigue and Immune Dysfunction Syndrome (CFIDS), a complex illness associated with low-level radiation exposure. In the Covidıg pandemic age, I am also addressing those of you who survived Covidıg but still suffer lingering effects. You are known as long-haulers, and I feel for you as I suffered the same way with a post-viral fatigue myself. Many doctors do not believe that the effects of Covidıg can still exist and fail to give you any medication for lingering effects. Viruses sometimes leave a signature behind or hide inside the spinal cord. In the first case, we call it a post-viral syndrome, which needs to follow its own time schedule to disappear. An example of a virus hiding in the spinal cord would be the chicken pox, *varicella* virus. We can have the illness in childhood and then as adults; it returns in a very different and painful disease called *shingles. Epstein Barr* virus is another example of a virus that presents as *mononucleosis*. It can then go into hiding and return when under stress in some cases of chronic fatigue syndrome.

Each illness has its own road on which to travel, but the journeys have some places in common. Most often, we need to change our lifestyle, or it is forced on us. We take medication and perhaps are forced to exercise to maintain muscle mass. I'm sure some of you reading this are very familiar with the nasty side effects of medications. Did your doctor prescribe steroids causing you to retain fluid? Does chemotherapy destroy your appetite giving you sores in your mouth and making you lose weight, especially muscle? Are you taking an NSAID (non-steroid anti-inflammatory drugs) such as *Advil*, putting your GI tract at risk for ulcers? Then when you develop the symptoms of ulcers, the doctor prescribes another medicine to counteract the side effects. Why must you suffer from the harmful effects of extra medications when there are foods you can eat that will eliminate the side effects!?

Eating foods dense in nutrients, enhances wellbeing; increases energy; helps us think more clearly; and provides the edge over other illness that might creep up from the long-term use of some medicines. Steroids, for example, come with a number of side effects. Doctors prescribe them for a variety of reasons, from stubborn rashes all the way to inflamed bowels, joints, and many autoimmune conditions. For the long-haulers, reading this, you may have been given this to keep your blood pressure up and mitigate the dizziness. However, this class of medicine puts us at risk of losing the main component of our bones: calcium. Even if you are using the inhaled form of a steroid, found in some inhalers, you could be losing calcium, putting you at risk for the bone-thinning disease, *osteoporosis*. The key to your bones' surviving this high-risk medication is to consistently increase the consumption of foods high in minerals and vitamins to keep the calcium where it belongs, inside the bones, and take the calcium supplements our health care provider recommends.

Imagine having the stamina to participate in that evening show that you've been wishing you had the energy to attend. Some of the most dangerous drugs on the market are biological response modifiers, (Humira, Rituxan, Remicade or Herceptin) which many people with rheumatoid arthritis, IBD, or some skin conditions are given. These are also used in cancer therapy. And yes, they can produce miraculous improvement. However, just like every drug, there's a downside: their use increases the risk of many other diseases besides osteoporosis. Even the Flu could become a major risk to your health as these medications turn off the protective mechanisms our immune system uses to hunt down invading organisms. Wouldn't it be empowering if you could prevent other illnesses while *enjoying* a diet that promotes a strong, vital immune system!

If you were diagnosed with heart disease and taking diuretic pills, you might not need them as often if you follow a diet naturally rich in the minerals that keep blood pressure from skyrocketing. Imagine saying good bye to those pills! Of course, you need to do this with your doctor on board. Eating foods that keep inflammation at bay may also prevent the disease from occurring from the very start.

HIDDEN INFLAMERS

We think of bread as the "Staff of life." However, for many of us with chronic illness, the GI tract may not work as efficiently as it once did. Did you know that the bread we eat can CAUSE inflammation, joint aches, brain fog, and weakness if you are one of the thousands of people that have developed an intolerance to the higher gluten flour used in commercial bread baking? I will provide you with an eating plan that does not rely heavily on wheat.

Feeling stronger, empowered, and more knowledgeable about your body is within your grasp. Even with obstacles in your path, you can embrace change with an open mind. I know you chose this book because you are too damned tired to cook, or the thought of creating a meal, sends you to the couch. But you can still eat in ways that will energize you and help you sleep more soundly while building up your immune system, even if you don't know the difference between a crock pot and a chafing dish.

This book gives the tools you need to nourish your body while guiding you along the path to increased vitality. First, you may like to learn about my path and what brought me to writing this book.

THE MONO THAT WASN'T

One hot summer's day I started to experience unbelievable fatigue. In addition, my throat was sore, my ears ached, my liver was tender, and I lost my appetite. My doctors thought I had Mononucleosis except the mono-spot came back negative. Doctors have a more descriptive name for the sore red throat, referring to it as the "crimson crescents." To me, it felt as I had accidentally inhaled the entire wad of cotton that comes packed inside a bottle of aspirin and it felt as though half of the wad was hanging down in the back of my throat. I found it difficult to concentrate and couldn't comprehend what I read. The words swam across the page, losing all meaning. Two months later came emergency room visits with chest pain diagnosed as *"Costo-chondritis"* a painful, yet harmless irritation of the cartilage in my chest wall, as well as severe back pain. My neck hurt repeatedly, and my head felt too heavy to hold up. I felt dizzy all the time and had minimal appetite. Many specialists ran more tests, but no one illness could be diagnosed, even though the symptoms continued to linger.

Thus began a year of doctor appointments, physical therapy visits, seeing a chiropractor for the first time, and resting in bed the rest of the time. It was the onset of my CFIDS, yet I did not know it and would not receive that diagnosis until *years* later. Tests followed, including X-rays, MRIs, and CT scans that showed orthopedic problems but nothing which could account for the exhaustion and infections. My doctors told me that the amount of pain I experienced did not match up with the findings on their scans. A year or two later, came a diagnosis of Fibromyalgia (FM). All the doctors could tell me was that it would not progress and become worse, but I would need physical therapy to strengthen me. One physical therapist explained that my muscles had a fibrous covering all over them, much like "Spiderman" that needed to be released through massage and ultrasound treatments.

FROM THIS DAY FORWARD

I was referred to a rehabilitation hospital where I met with my physiatrist, Dr. "X." Physiatrists practice 'physical medicine', which to me is an expanded version of physical therapy (PT) with the addition of painful procedures such as nerve blocks. If the PT's are unable to get a muscle to stretch adequately, they use "Spray n Stretch" to numb the pain and send you back to the doctor for an additional round of torture. Would you believe Dr. "X" would park his motorcycle in the lobby of the hospital, placing his black shiny rider's helmet on the office desk? I don't know what you do, about motorcycles, but ER doctors refer to them as "donor cycles." I guess Dr. "X" considered himself to be invincible.

Rehab hospitals deal with severely damaged brains and spinal cords, and they offer the treatment of serious diseases such as *multiple sclerosis* and *muscular dystrophy*, employing many physiatrists, neurologists, and even social workers on staff. Despite its cheerfully painted framed pictures of wild birds in the outpatient waiting room, I felt only pain and despair seeping out of every wall. One day, a very young neurologist came at me with a pin, which he literally poked completely through my skin, starting from my head downward, to check my sensation; I won't choose that from the menu of tortures ever again.

I had left the safety of my local hospital where I knew everyone and entered the inner sanctum of a place where patients routinely undergo painful tests and procedures in order to deal with conditions that tear their lives apart. Did I really need to undergo various forms of torture wearing nothing more than a cotton gown in order to become well?

THE ANGEL INTERVENES

I endured outpatient hospital visits two or three times per week to receive physical therapy (manual stretching) techniques for my neck, which aggravated my sensitivity to light and increased the severity of my headaches. In addition to this, I joined a gentle yoga class near my house. Six weeks into a class where at first we reclined on the floor to do some mild stretching, I could move normally. I didn't realize my yoga instructor, Pat, spoke with my doctor. She gave the doctor a progress report one day on my range of motion, and I was gratefully discharged from his care. The day Angel Pat told me that I would N-E-V-E-R need to see that rehab facility ever again, lies indelibly etched in my memory. That meant no more forcing spoonfuls of Benadryl down my throat, to endure that nauseating car ride to reach the rehab. No more hours of sitting in the waiting room surrounded by all those walkers and canes, oxygen tanks, and wheelchairs. Was I cured? No, but my "head bone" was once again connected to my "neck bone" and I had functional strength in my muscles. My other doctors would monitor my progress from thereon.

Doctor visits continued, I learned how to hunt down waiting rooms that had soft lighting rather than the glare of fluorescent lights. When things were really bad with my photophobia—that's 'the medical term for eyes being sensitive to light—I walked into an exam room and turned off the lights, while waiting to be seen. Some doctors actually didn't turn the lights back on. Nothing kinky; they just realized how severe my pain was and made do with the light from the hall to conduct their exams.

Even though I had a wonderful primary care doctor, the now deceased and much-loved, Dr, Guillermo Asis, who was also a specialist in Chronic Fatigue Syndrome, it was a challenge to get to his office. I had to stand on a train platform for up to 20 minutes and change to a trolley to get to his Brookline office, especially when I was unable to obtain a seat during any part of the ride through the Boston subway. Since I did not fit the categories of pregnant or elderly, even though I felt ninety years old, I had no choice but to stand for the thirty-minute ride and pray that I did not pass out on the way there. I'd feel myself growing weaker and weaker as I approached my destination. Once inside the waiting room office, with the fervency of a bloodhound to find a lost child, I sought out a sofa to collapse on. If the waiting room didn't have a sofa on which to lie, I found two arm-less chairs, placing two or more together to fit my small frame. I didn't yet know that a subset of people with CFIDS maintains only two-thirds of the rest of the population's blood volume. This lack of blood volume causes a corresponding decrease in blood pressure, making it difficult to stay erect and conscious.

Monthly sinus and ear infections arrived, making it seem as though I had a cold that would never leave. With this, I embarked on an unknown journey to try anything that would help me achieve normalcy. I wanted to be able to sit through a movie, join my friends at the mall, return to dance class, and to get my life back. Half of my monthly infections were treated visiting the local walk-in clinics, which only required a ten-minute bus ride. The down side of this is that you don't get seen by the same doctor each time, and no-one really follows your progress. Back in the 1990's the criteria to diagnose what was then called Chronic Fatigue Syndrome, involved incurring a new infection each month for six consecutive months. If I had only dragged myself into one doctor's office instead of several, I *might* have been diagnosed with CFIDS sooner. At the time, neither FM nor CFS had any established treatment, so I did not realize I was doing myself any disservice.

I needed a team of people to help me in my recovery to battle the exhaustion, pain, and new symptoms that frighteningly appeared by the week. Traditional medical doctors gave me antibiotics for my ear infections and strep throats. Nutritionists helped me sort out food intolerances and allergies and helped me to strengthen my immune system. Too often, I was intolerant of the treatments. I'd pick up a prescription for an antibiotic and end up in the Emergency room from reactions to it. It was so discouraging to purchase three bottles of supplements at $30 apiece and not be able to tolerate them. Many made me dizzy and I got excruciating headaches from others. My friends and family believed I had become a hypochondriac. Even I began to suspect the same as life revolved around sickness and the regimens I needed to follow to get well.

As is typical for a person with CFIDS or FM, I would visit the doctor to find out I had not just one but two infections simultaneously. Part of the course of my illness was to have strep throat and bronchitis one week and an ear infection with infected sinuses the next. Out of one box into another I'd walk from the medical center to the drugstore nearby. I used to feel so horribly dizzy standing in line at the pharmacy, feeling like a character from the Zombie Apocalypse movie.

THANK GOODNESS FOR SUPPORT GROUPS

I remember one day my dear mother found a small advertisement in the local paper for a support group for Chronic Fatigue Syndrome/Fibromyalgia. These precious meetings, started sprouting up in the Boston area. Attending, I listened to others coping with these two awful conditions, finding great dissonance between what the media reported about the disease, which they said affected "couch potatoes," and the flesh and blood people in my support groups. These people were avid bicyclists, mountain hikers, and dancers suddenly struck down by an invisible illness and BECAME "couch potatoes." At one support meeting, a man described how tiring it was to make a peanut butter and jelly sandwich. By the time he had spread the peanut butter on one slice of bread, he needed to lie down before he could manage to put the jelly on the other slice. I considered myself lucky that this was not me, but was soon in for a shock when I experienced my first relapse.

People far more advanced along the illness spectrum attended support group meetings accompanied by different paraphernalia, including those dreaded oxygen tanks which I felt helpless to avoid. Would I be on oxygen support in a few years? It was not uncommon for people to bring a bedroom pillow and lie on the floor for the meeting duration. There was a dimmer switch in the room where we met with the lights always turned down low to accommodate the light sensitivity from which many of us suffer.

Within a group of people as achy as me, with enlarged and painful lymph glands, and toting water bottles everywhere to replace the lost fluid volume, I finally found the strange planet where I belonged. I looked forward to attending the monthly support group meeting where medical journal articles were shared and interpreted. The attendees related their experiences, good or bad, with health practitioners.

Every once in a while, a brave journalist would relay her experience of living with CFS in a magazine article. After reading one woman's journey with CFS treated with TCM (Traditional Chinese Medicine), I visited a Chinese medical practitioner with an open mind. To my surprise, I was not sent home with a bag of twigs and leaves to boil into a concoction as the journalist had. It was much more straightforward. All of the herbal remedies I was given resembled BB shots, except they were either black or maroon rather than gunmetal gray in color. You take them with a glass of warm water, the doctor encouraging me to try it in front of him before I left. It was the first time I ever drank water that was warm, not hot, so soothing to my inflamed mucous membranes, and it relaxed all of the tight muscles in my throat. From there on, I added warm water to my hydration regimen, adopting my grandmother's weird practice of drinking warm water.

It was onto homeopathic medicine which felt like "voodoo" to someone trained in Nutrition at Simmons College, so steeped in traditional methodology that Harvard Medical School faculty provided some of the lectures. Homeopathy is a most unusual system, following a theory of "like" cures "like." You are given such a tiny dilution of a substance that really only the "energy" of the substance is present to bring on symptoms to eliminate them. Unusual things are used, including seeds, shells, feathers, and venom. All were provided to me in tiny, white uniform-sized balls the doctor placed under my tongue for the first dose. I was given Cocculus for motion sickness and Rhus tox for pain. Some things worked and some things didn't have any effect.

Chronic Fatigue Syndrome, now referred to as SEID or Systemic Exertion Intolerance Syndrome, doesn't sound like an accurate name for a condition that involves a dysfunctional immune system. People with this illness have deficient amounts of natural killer cells (NK). Due to the deficient amount, these killer cells are unable to do their important job of surveilling and destroying invading organisms such as bacteria, viruses, and fungi. Parts of the immune system are hyper-responsive, reacting to foods, medications, and environmental triggers. In contrast, other parts lack the vigilance they need, so a person with this will catch every 'bug" going around. I vividly remember my doctor telling me that I was like a 'walking petri dish', as I contracted every viral and bacterial infection that came my way.

As we react to invading organisms, our bodies produce hormones called *"cytokines,"* flooding the bloodstream and creating the low-grade fevers characteristic of the illness with resulting aches all over. Many other conditions have this in common, even people undergoing cancer chemotherapy. The chemo, in this case causes the body to release the cytokines. This cytokine release also makes people with the Flu feel like a fourteen-wheeler ran them over. And the cytokine "storm" is what is killing some people with Covid19. The body launches an all-out attack against the virus, unfortunately killing the person with it.

The National Academy of Sciences, a branch of the National Institute of Health (NIH), has come out with DRI's or Daily recommended Intakes of nutrients, which take the place of what some of you may remember as Recommended Dietary allowances. The daily values of the DRI are written for healthy people and are judged inadequate for many. Anyone fighting any chronic illness or the after-effects of a virus such as Covid19, has a weakened body and needs super-nutrition to heal the damaged tissues.

My biggest challenge through the worst years of my illness has been feeding myself. With such utter exhaustion, putting together a healthy meal often presents a huge challenge, despite my nutrition knowledge. I realized then how much more difficult it must be for the person without any formal training in nutrition to obtain adequate nutrients while contending with both pain and weakness, and that is how I came to write this book. I know what it is like to be so tired that you literally fall asleep on your dinner plate. I have experienced weakness and low blood pressure so severe that I needed to lie down on the bench at the commuter rail station, looking like a homeless person lying there.

This book will help those journeying through chronic illness through good nutrition, which is the cornerstone of a healthier life, to become stronger and more resilient to other diseases. When an illness weakens our bodies, we need strong defenses to fight back. A diet loaded with anti-oxidant rich foods will arm us with the tools we need to remain standing. We need foods packed with minerals and vitamins in their natural state, not from a package, to replenish lost stores, fortify energy systems, and repair damaged tissues. Improving the quality of our diet can help heal the GI tract, increasing the healthy bacteria we need to boost our immune system, lower unhealthy cholesterol, and blood pressure, or normalize a metabolism that may have slowed down to a crawl, so that we can have the edge over diseases such as cancer, heart disease, diabetes, and others.

CHAPTER 2

FROZEN, TAKE-OUT AND READY TO EAT

You know those days when you barely have the time (or energy) to cook a meal. Maybe you've just returned home from the afternoon parent-teacher conference where surprise! Your little cherub is failing in math. You really don't want to spend the evening poring over his math assignments with him. It's the last thing you want to do. After a full day's work, you might be irritable and finding it difficult to stay focused. Now it's 4 p.m. and you need to get supper started, and you forgot to defrost the meat for tonight. At times like these, take-out food can become a viable solution with just a few tweaks.

Many of the courses from the Asian culture are full of attractive and good-for-you vegetables. In-fact, crunchy stir-fried vegetables are a staple of Chinese food. If you make the right choices, Chinese food can be healthy when you skip the batter-fried and deep-fried items. Choose the meat and shrimp dishes full of dark green leafy vegetables. I'm going to coin a new term for the broccoli, Bok choy, and spinach, all loaded with antioxidants and cancer preventing goodies such as heart healthy, Folate. I am going to refer to them as the "leafies." The best part about take-out Chinese food is all the chopping and slicing is done for you!

Let me explain why anti-oxidants in their natural state as whole foods (not from supplements) are so crucial. In order to gain energy from the foods we eat, food needs to be "burned," which means combined with oxygen. Unfortunately, this reaction, referred to by scientists as "oxidation" analogous to rust accumulating on a piece of iron, generates by-products that damage cells. Anti-oxidants prevent this build-up at the cellular level and accelerate the death of abnormal cells from toxins such as environmental pollution, tobacco, radiation, including the amount we get from our cell phones, tablets, and computers, as well as infection.

Both *Lo mein* and *Chow mein* feature bean sprouts and celery. To bring this dish to an amazing nutritional level, just add a bag of frozen broccoli crowns or another cruciferous vegetable such as cauliflower. They steam nicely in very little water. These are full of sulfur-containing compounds that protect all our cells from developing cancerous tumors.

If you don't have a tasty Asian sauce available, a tangy squirt of lemon from one of those little plastic lemons enhances flavor in a pinch. Both Whole Foods and Trader Joe stores sell these free of the sulfite preservative many of us with chronic illness may react to. Why is sulfite used in the first place? It keeps foods such as apples and potatoes from turning brown. Anyone with asthma or a respiratory condition, may be advised to avoid sulfites linked to the narrowing of airways, in some cases leading to full-blown attacks.

Chinese entrees celebrate the use of Napa cabbage or Bok Choy, both of which are in the same cruciferous family as broccoli. The oil used to stir-fry Chinese food is often healthy peanut or sesame oil. When you place your order, request entrees of beef, chicken, pork, fish, or tofu. With so much of the population now sensitive to the flavor-enhancer, *monosodium glutamate* (MSG), many Chinese restaurants cook without this substance, which gives many of us headaches. Request the brown rice if they have it. More Chinese restaurants make brown rice available, which boosts our fiber intake while providing us Magnesium.

THAI AND VIETNAMESE FOOD

Another Asian cuisine I embrace is Thai. Seasoned with coconut and peanut sauce, Thai food features rice or noodles as well as wide rice noodles in combo with beef, chicken, seafood, or tofu. While the Chinese feature soy, garlic, and ginger, Thai spices include curry, basil, and lemongrass. The crucifers play less of a feature than in Chinese food. Something as ordinary as carrots or green beans will be spiced up with an aromatic blend of Thai Basil and sliced in very creative ways on your plate.

I'm so lucky to live in the North East, where a veritable melting pot of foods surround me. Thai, Vietnamese, Korean. All are good choices. Far better for me than the hamburgers and French fries offered in most American food restaurants.

I enjoy Vietnamese food now because I know how to navigate my way around the menus. However, during my first visit to a Vietnamese restaurant, I walked out with an empty stomach, and a burnt tongue as the food was fiery-hot. I've since learned that milder foods exist on the menu, and I may always request that "no spice" be used. Yes, those magical words make a world of difference! The dish, Bee Boing, consist of a trio of soft rice noodles, cucumbers, and bean sprouts in a dressing of coconut milk and peanut sauce, dusted with mint leaves. It can be ordered with pork, shrimp, or chicken. *Pho* soup, hearty and nourishing broth with vegetables, rice noodles, bean sprouts and Basil leaves, can be ordered in either wheat or rice noodle versions with Beef or Chicken.

Healthy options abound from these menus. Often plain old iceberg lettuce is served on the plate with the meat and vegetables. Other restaurants will use healthier romaine lettuce. I like *Ban Hoi*. In this dish, soft rice noodles, bean sprouts, mint leaves, and cucumbers are drenched in a savory peanut sauce and served alongside a half plate of garden-fresh Bibb lettuce. You fold the ingredients into the leaves and roll them yourself at the table. This can also be ordered with shrimp, chicken, or pork. Noodle bowls can be made of rice or wheat noodles and cucumbers.

Korean dishes use meat and fish and feature eggs and lots of colorful veggies. One I am fond of is *Bitumibab*. This is cooked carrots, sprouts, mushrooms, strips of romaine lettuce, rice, and an egg, usually nestled in the center of the dish. The addition of meat to this dish is optional. I was pleased when I found this offered on the menu of a lunch place in town. Be sure to ask for the un-spicy version if you are not into spicy foods. Koreans feature fermented cabbage dishes in the form of *kimchi*. These are tasty cabbage side-dishes often served with fruit mixed in with the cabbage. Kimchi is cultured cabbage and provides pro-biotic benefits which you can find in your Whole Foods Store.

THE BRAZILIAN BUFFET

For a nutritionist walking into a Brazilian buffet is like entering into food heaven. Not only is the food hot and mouthwateringly delicious, but you don't even need to wait for a waiter to come to your table to serve you. The quantity of fresh vegetables is incredible! The typical Brazilian buffet featuring a delectable assortment of rice, potatoes, as well as beans dusted with yucca flour - which looks like bread crumbs. You'll see broccoli, carrots, cauliflower, onions, red peppers, tomatoes and usually two kinds of fruit such as kiwi and melons. A separate station for meat includes choices of beef, chicken, and sausage. The food is always very colorful and appealing, and the vegetables are never over cooked.

Be aware of the tempting dessert case, which often sits beside the cash register full of delectable cakes, tarts, and pies, which are okay in moderation. The beverages include mango, papaya, guava, and almond juices, and strong coffee and tea.

Brazilian buffets vary in their policies. At some, you pay a flat fee for all-you-can- eat. At others, you pay by the weight. Save room on your plate for the meat. It is carved right at the carving station hot off the spit. In some Brazilian restaurants, the meat is brought to the table on long metal skewers, which you slide with a fork onto your plate. Brazilians make it a cinch to eat your five servings of fruit and vegetables in just one delicious meal! But I don't recommend this unless you are used to eating this amount of fiber. If you don't currently eat this amount of fruit and vegetables at one time, it could cause intestinal distress. I've counseled some clients who come to me, eating only five fruits and vegetables in a week, let alone one meal! So, work up to eating five servings of produce in one delicious meal.

PLANNING MEALS

Who plans meals? Hardly anyone wants to do it. You'd be surprised how many people never come up with a plan for eating. Oh, everyone does this when you are hosting a party. You painstakingly plan the menu and shop for all the ingredients but for the majority, planning a week's menus is avoided, much like going to the dentist.

Getting a meal may consist of a hurried forage through the fridge and cabinets, missing things that have traveled to the back of the refrigerator, never to be seen again. Meal planning should not be a painful chore. Sure, it is stressful to plan a meal when you are hurtling down the aisles of the supermarket, with one child riding in the front of the carriage and the other balancing on the back with only half an hour until dinnertime. Let's consider something more restful and deliberate.

I actually plan my meals lying down on my sofa. I just close my eyes, taking a few deep breaths to center myself, shutting out all the distractions (no TV, no Facebook, and the cell phone is shut off) to reach a more mellow place. Now from this relaxed centered place, consider what you would really like to eat, which is also good for your body.

This is how you plan your meals and your shopping list. Sit or lie in a comfortable place with a pen and a sheet of paper. If you are like most people, and you tend to reach out for foods with a creamy consistency such as ice cream when you feel stressed, why not substitute some Greek yogurt with honey? This also provides that creamy and smooth texture. Some Greek yogurts have the surprisingly seductive consistency of cheese cake—without containing all the calories that a wedge of cheesecake supplies. You can satisfy your taste buds as well as your blood sugar by indulging in this high protein snack food. Creamy polenta with spinach and carrots is another comfort food. Thanks to Trader Joe's frozen food aisle, this dinner time treat comes in a plastic bag, and all you need to do is open the bag and heat it with a little bit of water.

Throughout my journey with chronic fatigue, appetite has been a problem. Those of you undergoing radiation treatments, chemotherapy, or just suffering from a cold probably don't have much of one, especially if you have sores inside your mouth and on your tongue. Many of you with "long haulers" may have lost your sense of taste and smell, making it even harder to eat. Some chicken soup might appeal to you. Associated not only with comfort, mothers for centuries, have fed their loved one varieties of a broth made from chicken or even duck. Researchers from major universities studied the components in chicken broth, and found they actually provide a physical benefit—they loosen nasal secretions.[1] (That's welcome news for those of with stuffed up noses or even chronic sinus problems.) Chicken soup is powerful medicine acting as a natural antibiotic as well as decongestant. The *carnosine* formed when chicken and vegetables merge actually kills viruses.[2] Some of you may have reduced your intake of wheat products for various reasons and prefer to add some gluten-free pasta or quick-cooking barley to your broths. The little tan-colored nuggets of barley are easy on the stomach while thickening the broth, and as a bonus, they provide iron and folate, both important nutrients for our immune systems.

MORE ABOUT SOUPS AND CHICKEN

As our society became aware of the excessive amount of sodium found in canned soups, manufacturers offered lower sodium soups, substituting sea salt and compounds such as potassium chloride in place of table salt. If you are diagnosed with high blood pressure,

---

[1] Rennard, B.O., Ertl R.F., Gossman, G.L., Robbins, R.A., & Rennard, S.I. (2000). Chicken soup inhibits neutrophil chemotaxis in vitro. *Chest*, 118(4), 1150-1157.

[2] Babizhayev, MA, Deyev, AI, and Yegorov, YE. Non-hydrolyzed in digestive tract and blood natural L-carnosine peptide ("bioactivated Jewish Penicillin") as a panacea of tomorrow for various flu ailments: signaling activity attenuating nitric oxide (NO) production, cytostasis, and NO-dependent inhibitor of influenza virus replication in macrophage in the human body infected with the virulent swine influenza A (H1N1) virus. *Journal of Basic and Clinical Physiology and Pharmacology*, 24(1), 1-26.

these may be helpful. Some of us with SEID or Fibromyalgia, may be suffering from a completely different problem: low blood pressure. In this case, your health care provider may have advised you to add salt. Then you need to avoid those soups made with potassium chloride. One thing we all need to avoid is preservatives. They make food last longer on the shelves but damage our health. You can find soups without preservatives in the brands, *Imagine* and *Pacific* and a few organic Trader Joe soups sold in cartons, and the healthier product lines sold in Stop and Shop (Nature's Promise) and Shaws (Nature's Way) in my region. All your favorites come in cartons now: beef, vegetable, and chicken broths. Creamy soups such as carrot-ginger, mushroom, tomato and roasted pepper/tomato can easily be used as the foundation of a meal by adding a cooked grain and a leafy green vegetable which doesn't always need to be cooked. Try a handful of arugulas or a few leaves of romaine lettuce added to the pot just before serving.

Lettuce, with the exception of nutritionally-impoverished iceberg, is rich in minerals, magnesium, and calcium that allow muscles to contract and relax with ease. If the soup you choose is low in protein, (3 grams or less), simply toss in some chicken, pork, or beef cooked from a previous meal. For a vegetarian boost, add cooked legumes such as chick peas to the pot. Just rinse canned beans well under cool, running water to eliminate most of the salt.

In my first manuscript for this book, I suggested using canned chicken. Although the dangers of plastic liners in canned foods have been acknowledged, I'm waiting for the manufacturers to stop using BPA liners so that I'm not getting nasty *Bis-phenol A* that gets absorbed into my food. BPA is a chemical used in the plastic liners of most cans and some bottles. Research now links it to serious problems with the reproductive and endocrine systems in children and heart disease in adults.[3] For those of you not concerned about BPA, read all canned food labels carefully to ensure that the cans of chicken are clearly 100% chicken and not filled with soy protein as filler. Many cans of chicken and tuna are often packed with soy as filler, which I like to avoid. Approximately two years ago, I was served some pretty bad-tasting tuna at a relative's home. When we checked the can, we found the "tuna" was never tuna but textured soy protein. So be sure to check those tuna fish labels!!

You might ask, 'What's wrong with soy? Isn't soy supposed to be good for me?' Unprocessed forms of soy are beneficial, with fermented forms being the best. Studies show that Asian women rarely develop breast cancer or any other cancer from their consumption of non-genetically modified (non-GMO) tofu soy, which undergoes barely any processing. However, the highly processed textured soy protein used as a filler in some canned chicken and soy products, as well as in plant-based burgers and sausages, in this country, is far from healthy! The way we grow soy in the United States gained attention from other countries when the entire European Union refused to accept any American exports of our genetically modified soy.

IT'S OK TO SLURP

A good quality soup can be chosen as a snack or even form the basis of a meal. Check the label for its fiber content because that fiber keeps us full. Eating a cup of soup keeps me from becoming hungry two hours after a meal. On the other hand, I can make a meal with

---

[3] Melzer, D., Rice, N.E., Lewis, C., Henley, W.E., & Galloway, T.S. (2010). Association of urinary bisphenol a concentration with heart disease: evidence from NHANES 2003/06. *PloS one*, 5(1), e8673.

a package of bean soup in 10 minutes, simply adding it to a leftover grain (brown rice, whole-wheat couscous, or cooked quinoa.) Don't forget to add those all-important leafy greens! The NCI (National Cancer Institute) now recommends that everyone consume at least one leafy green vegetable every day for their excellent anti-oxidant protection.

There is nothing simpler to use than baby spinach, washed and drained or frozen. I've organized a few soup and green/grain combinations in this chart. Keep reading to find out the secret of why these are so healthy.

A MEAL MADE FROM CREAMY SOUP

Start with a Soup	Add a Grain	. . . and a Green	Finish with a Protein
carrot ginger	soft corn tortilla	romaine lettuce	diced chicken
mushroom	quick cooking barley	European blend	1 oz. of hard cheese
tomato	whole wheat couscous	arugula	canned wild salmon
corn chowder	sprouted wheat bread	baby spinach	deli bean salad
butternut squash	instant brown rice	red leaf lettuce	crumbled feta cheese

Because these are vegetable-based soups, they are not high in protein. But you can choose bean soups, which boast 4 grams of protein per serving. If this leaves you hungry, you can always add more. In the table above, I've added an extra column of ideas. Bean soups are just begging to have some colorful greens added to them. You can eat your greens as a side dish or just stir them into the soup as it heats. And the lunch meal would not be balanced without a piece of fruit to quench thirst, plus add additional vitamins and minerals along with color and antioxidants.

A MEAL FROM A BEAN-BASED SOUP

Start with a Soup	Add a Green	A Piece of Fruit	Other Protein
Amy's black beans and rice	spinach	apple	pre-cooked shrimp
white bean soup	curly green lettuce	peach or apricot	deli roast beef
Dr. McDougall's split pea with barley	watercress	grapefruit or kiwi	handful of almonds
organic tortilla bean soup	broccoli	red grapes, strawberries	1 hard boiled egg

CREATING A LIST OF STAPLES

On a day when there are fewer disturbances, create for yourself a list of staples to have on hand. My own pantry holds an array of grains purchased from bulk bins at the health foods store: millet, quinoa, buckwheat, and amaranth sit in glass jars on shelves. There are days when I have the energy to cook a whole grain. I know that many of you may not yet have this stamina but for now, you can rely on instant grains to see you through. Some of the better choices to keep on our shelves include: instant brown rice, which has been parboiled; organic whole wheat couscous; and barley, all of which you heat in water or a broth. Purchase a bag of Bob's red mill *ground* flaxseed or chia seeds which you can add to cereals, soups, and salads to obtain their omega 3 benefits, which quell inflammation. But keep these in the fridge as they are perishable. And sweet potatoes and yams. I mention both because depending on where you live, one may be more available than the other. These potatoes are a cinch to make. Simply rinse the potato under running water, then stick the tines of a fork into it to allow for the gases to escape. Preheat oven to 425°F. Then pop them in for 45 minutes to 1 hour, depending on the size. You will see the sweet juices coming out of the holes you made. A pat of organic or grass-fed butter and some black pepper, completes this side dish.

NO MICROWAVE PLEASE

Most chronic illness symptoms go up and down like the NASDAQ with flares when facing an important event. This is when we are tempted to use the microwave oven. Although this makes cooking faster and easier, I noticed a dramatic DECREASE in my number of colds and infections when I started living without a microwave oven to cook my meals. Did you know that microwaves are not as safe as the manufacturers lead you to believe? Microwaves tend to alter the nutrients in food at a cellular level, destroying some nutrients. In most chronic illnesses, oxidation at the cellular level is speeded up, making us require more antioxidants than the rest of the population. Furthermore, the cell's energy factory, the mitochondria, are impacted by chronic illness, so greater care should be taken to preserve all the nutrients we take in. Our requirement for nutrients is higher than for people without illness.

In a study done at the Islamic University, corn seedlings were fed microwaved water, affecting the leaves' chlorophyll. In case you don't know, chlorophyll is the pigment that gives leaves their bright green color. We eat those green leafy vegetables to obtain all the nutrients inside them. However, microwaving alters the cell membrane, containing all the nutrients. So, DON'T use your microwave if you want to feel better!

Additionally, research dating back to October of 1994 found Salmonella, a bacteria we hear about constantly in the news, as a source of food poisoning, is not completely killed during the microwave process.[4,5,6,7] This is especially important to consider when handling undercooked and raw poultry and eggs.

WHAT TO KEEP ON HAND

By eating whole foods (the least processed), we harness our energy. Who has the stamina to stand over a hot stove, even for half an hour? Therefore, this book meets you where you are - at the low end of the energy scale. I will guide you through the use of take-out, frozen, and convenience foods made without artificial dyes and preservatives. I shall show you how to optimize your choices of these, and we will incorporate high fiber foods so we can get Super Energy. We will be stocking up on organic foods with their superior nutrient profile. In fact, I will emphasize organic food

---

[4] Culkin, KA and Fung, YC. Destruction of E. Col and Salmonella typhimurium in Microwave-cooked soups *Journal of Milk Food Technology.* Vol 38, No. 1 Pages 8-15, January 1975

[5] Fung, DYC & Cunningham, FE. (1980) 43(8): 641-650 Effect of Microwaves on Microorganisms in Foods. J. Food Prot. https://doi.org/10.4315/0362-028X-43.8.641

[6] Bates, C.J & and Spencer, R.C. Survival of Salmonella species in eggs poached using a microwave oven. *Journal of Hospital Infection, 29(2), 121-127.*

[7] http://www.lessemf.com/mw-stnds.html microwave oven radiation hazards & standards. US Food and Drug Administration, HHS1030.10

throughout this entire book because it truly is the best! A study was done on preschoolers fed an organic diet for two weeks and a conventional diet for another two weeks. The researchers tested the urine of the kids. Guess what; there were *metabolites*, a fancy name for breakdown products of pesticides in the kids' urine when they were eating the conventionally grown produce. I don't know about you, but I steer clear of pesticides in my food supply. And you certainly don't want poisons lurking in your child's body!

You don't want to make too many trips to the grocery store. It sure is not a fun way to spend the day, so choose foods with a longer shelf life: apples, lemons, sweet potatoes, onions, garlic, and white potatoes. You'll also want to have a package of frozen onions and a jar of minced garlic in oil for flavor. Onions and garlic have awesome antioxidant activity! They contain sulfur to boost immune function; therefore, I use them daily. When I had a sore throat, my natural doctor had me eat a raw garlic clove every day. Whoa! You say, "I'm not doing that!' Exactly what I thought. However, I figured out a way to get it in. I opened a can of chicken and squeezed the garlic clove through my handy-dandy garlic press. I spread it on bread with a tiny bit of mayo, salt, and pepper. I ate it open-faced and, to my amazement, it actually tasted great! And I got relief from the sore throat for four full hours! Garlic also acts as a protector against cancer-causing substances, and onions, (red and yellow), contain *quercetin*, which assists the immune system. Flavonoids in onions strengthen blood vessel walls.

You'll also want to have these staples in the house: quick-cooking whole grains such as oatmeal, quinoa flakes, which cook in a minute and half; whole wheat couscous; instant brown rice; and some pasta that supplies 3 grams of fiber per serving.

When you walk down the pasta aisle, it's no longer just blue and yellow boxes of durum wheat. It's a very colorful place now with red boxes of red lentil pasta, yellow boxes of protein-enriched pasta, and others. Expand your world to varieties made from gluten-free flours: rice, corn, quinoa, millet, even lentil beans, and chickpea flour! These often provide 3 to 4 grams of fiber for every serving, a serving being 3/4 cup. Whereas ordinary pasta does not. Remember, the fiber keeps us feeling full longer, so we are not sneaking into the kitchen to eat snickerdoodles at 2 a.m. You may have noticed I did not mention Whole Wheat Pasta. There is a reason for this to come.

You can read more about pasta in chapter 9. You also want to stock your pantry and cupboard with Extra Virgin Olive Oil (EVOO), which is the oil least likely to cause inflammation in our bodies. This versatile and healthy oil can be used on salads, on top of vegetables in place of butter, for cooking on low heat, and even as a delicious dip for breads.

CHAPTER 3

MORE UNPROCESSED GRAINS

I hope that you are not wedded to those little puffed up grains of white rice and corn in the form of convenience cereals. These are so refined that there isn't much left in them other than a puff of air. They lack the nutrients and fiber or roughage we need leaving us hungry!

Roughage is like the personal trainer inside our intestines, ensuring they exercise by having adequate fiber, and helping us avoid cravings for unhealthy foods.

We need to start eating WHOLE grains as they are loaded with minerals and vitamins, especially zinc, because of its much-needed importance for our immune systems. According to a review study done by Polish researchers, zinc-rich foods keep bodies from breaking down testosterone,[8] needed for reproductive health and

---

[8] Nasiodek, M., Stragierrwicz, J. M. Klimozak, M., & Kilanowicz, A.(2020) The role of zinc in selected female reproductive disorders. Nutrients 12(8), 2464. https://doi.org/10.3390/nu12082464

both females and males. In addition, two energy Vitamins, B1 and B2 are both found in whole grain foods.

Do you want to reduce your risk of type 2 diabetes? Whole grains can help you work toward accomplishing that as well![9]

Let's compare a cup of white rice to brown rice:

White Rice	Brown Rice
little satiety	greater satiety
0.6 grams of fiber	3.5 grams of fiber
57 mg. of Potassium	137 mg. of Potassium
19 mg. of Magnesium	36 mg of Magnesium
no lignans	high in lignans
drives up blood sugar	keeps blood sugar stable
242 Kcal	218 Kcal
1/2 amount of Manganese	double the amount of Manganese

For those with fluid retention problems, potassium can be the missing component you need to get rid of the excess fluid. This mineral also helps the heart maintain a steady beat. Compare brown rice's 137 mg of potassium to only 57 mg found in white rice.

---

[9] Fung, T.T., Hu. F.B., Pereira, M.A., Liu, S., Stampfer, M.J., Colditz, G.A., & Willett, W.C. (2002) Whole-grain intake and the risk of type 2 diabetes: a prospective study in men. The American journal of clinical nutrition, 76(3), 535-540.

Potassium plays an important role in the health of our adrenal glands which work extra hard under the stress of chronic illness. Now, if you are worried about the research telling us that brown rice has more arsenic than white rice, don't worry too much because all you need to do is rinse the brown rice before cooking it.

DID YOU KNOW...

Brown rice is not a different type of rice? It comes from the same plant as white rice but still has all the nutritious parts intact.

MULTI-GRAIN IS *NOT* WHOLE

A friend of mine used to buy a multigrain bagel every morning, proudly believing she was eating whole grains for breakfast. The nutritionist in me had to inform her she was being fooled. Don't be hoodwinked by some of the words on bread packages, such as "multi-grain." You could be holding a loaf of bleached-out, overly processed grains, and the "multi" simply means more than one type of grain went into it: a bit of barley, mostly wheat, some millet perhaps, stripped of their healthy bran and the entire package of the multi-grain bread may contain zero grams of fiber!

Instead, look for these words: "whole wheat," "whole corn," "whole rye," "stone-ground corn," and "stone ground wheat" listed as the first and second ingredients on a package, and buy only organic corn products to avoid GMO's. Now my mission here, is to get you away from whole wheat products. They cause a host of inflammatory problems.

Have you tried the whole grain flatbreads and crisps such as *Suzie's Kamut* and spelt? These crisp breads are similar in texture to crackers yet full of fiber and low fat. Look for *Suzie's 7 Ancient Grain and Flax* flatbreads made with a variety of whole grains including *spelt*. For those of you unfamiliar with spelt, it is a form of wheat, (not yet subject as this book goes to press) to the genetic modifications plaguing regular wheat. You may want to try it for some variety and taste.

Another of my favorites is *Finn Crisp Rye breads* (the red box). These dark crunchy cracker-like breads are made of 100% rye flour and pair well with cheese (hard or soft). You will find crackers made of these as well. The old has become new again, regained popularity, as these flours don't have extra gluten added to them and have not been in the American food supply for too long. They are less likely to cause food intolerances. You may also find them easier to digest but they do contain some gluten. So, if you have Celiac, stay away from them! Pair any of these with cheese, soft goat cheese, or unsweetened apricot preserves. If you frequently experience stomach trouble, it may be time for you to experiment with more wheat-free foods. These are marketed for people with Celiac disease or those with gluten-intolerance, which are two different conditions. For example, the tapioca-based breads and crackers are not whole-grain, but they will offer you the same benefits as white bread while giving your GI tract a little rest time to allow the inflammation inside to subside.

CAUTION:

Wheat-free is not synonymous with gluten-free. People with Celiac Disease cannot tolerate wheat, barley, rye and sometimes oats. These grains containing Gluten have damaged their intestines, and every time they come into contact with gluten, it will continue to cause illness.

A growing set of the population is now becoming intolerant to the gluten in breads and pasta, available today. This may be due to the higher gluten content in these foods that was not present decades ago. Pick up a package of bread, and you will see the words "vital wheat gluten." Most people do not have an intestine adapted to consume this much gluten, and the immune system reacts with an allergic response to the gluten.

The healthy eating plan which I introduce in this book, limits wheat but does not restrict it altogether. I have much more energy by limiting wheat products and enjoy the gluten-free products available on supermarket shelves. A different type of wheat is found in spelt bread and here are two examples of spelt breads you will enjoy: *Rudi's Organic Spelt English muffins* and *Vermont Bread Company Spelt English muffins*. Now, for those who want gluten-free you may choose from several options, including *Canyon Bakehouse Heritage style bread* and *Rudi's*. Bread made using brown rice flour has a delicious texture and taste; you can find one that's refrigerated or frozen and Rudi's also sells GF tortillas and wrap breads. These are made with non-GMO ingredients and no high fructose corn syrup is used in any of Rudi's products. You find all of these in the freezer case. However, *Schär* has a line of breads and rolls that you will find on the shelf at room temperature rather than frozen, yet totally preservative-free.

BREAKFAST: REVVING YOUR ENGINE

Let's talk breakfast, the most important meal of the day, and the most often missed.

Did you know the word, 'Breakfast', literally means "break the fast"? Our bodies have been without food for 6-8 hours or more, depending on when the last meal or snack was eaten the night before. The proverbial, "tank" is empty, so we need to rev up our metabolic engines by putting food into our bodies. So make it QUALITY food! Now, I know, some of you wake up without any appetite and that's a problem we need to solve.

What happens to a person who doesn't eat a meal after waking up? Our body literally eats itself! Sounds like cannibalism, doesn't it? Our brains which need glucose (sugar) in order to work, have to obtain it from somewhere, so the liver does a process of breaking down food stores, to create glucose for our brains. If you have a few adipose deposits, these get used as fuel, but if you happen to be thin, your body will start to break down your muscle proteins in order to find a supply of food. I see this frequently at the gym, slender people whose bodies simply will not build muscle even though they lift weights regularly. Because they skip breakfast, their bodies consider them to be starving and use the protein that should normally build muscle, to fuel the brain instead. Our brains just happen to be the first priority for fuel assistance.

Now for those of you who are overweight, a slightly different process occurs. Your body starts to burn your fat storage as fuel, but in the process, *ketones* are produced, which are not designed to service our brains, and these are quite aromatic! You may work with someone who fasts frequently and tends to be irritable, anxious, dehydrated, and nauseous with difficulty concentrating. So maybe that bowl of whole grain cereal isn't looking so bad after all! We want to start the day with some protein and carbohydrate together in the right proportion; Greek yogurt with granola; cereal with grass fed milk in it plus another 8-ounce glass more; a hard-boiled egg with flatbreads and a piece of fruit. A two-ounce piece of cheese, with a handful of fresh strawberries and an organic granola bar. These are light breakfasts yet give us the fuel our bodies and brains crave to get through the morning. And if you feel like having a milk shake, choose an organic protein shake by Orgain. These are grass-fed and contain a hefty amount of protein, 26 grams, for every 14-ounce bottle. Protein foods take a bit longer to digest than the carbs, so they sustain us and keep us from becoming hungry.

HYPOGLYCEMIA - THE ROLLER COASTER OF BLOOD SUGAR

For many of us, a condition of hypoglycemia may accompany some of our other health problems. "Hypo" means "under" and "glycemic" refers to the sugar in our blood. The term then means our body doesn't have enough sugar to fuel our brains. Let's guess what symptoms can occur with this? Fuzzy thinking, as that poor brain is not getting the fuel it needs to calculate the percentage off that dress on sale at Macy's; blurry vision that gets in the way of what you are reading on Facebook; nausea or a sense of queasiness—certainly no real carnival ride. Some hypoglycemic conditions occur as a result of some medications. Other people are born with this condition. Still others develop it as a part of having Fibromyalgia and Chronic Fatigue, which involve the Adrenal gland not appropriately supported and creating wild fluctuations in blood sugar. I just hope that none of you are behind the wheel of a car driving with this untreated because you are an accident waiting to happen. Poor judgment and visual problems do not make a safe driver. Your health care provider can run blood sugar tests to find out if you have this.

The good news: the treatment is rather simple. You need to provide your body with protein at every meal and add two protein-filled snacks to your three meals. This condition is a popular one here in this country, so I have incorporated these principles into my eating plan I developed for you.

If you have hypoglycemia, the most important goal is to PREVENT your blood sugar from dropping. We want to keep it on an even keel. One way to do this is to eat whole grains, rather than the white kind. Only whole grains will slow down digestion to keep your blood sugar at a desirable level. In the case of wheat or corn, choose those with the USDA organic seal or symbol on the package to receive all the nutrients we need to equip our bodies with.

The USDA organic seal (usually placed on the front of the package), may be printed in brown and green or black and white, indicating that at least 95% of the product is organic. I emphasize organic so that you will receive the maximum amount of nutrients per serving. Unfortunately, mass- produced cereals from conventional farms, are grown in soil that lost most of its vitamins and minerals and won't provide enough nutrients.

Furthermore, pesticides and enormous amounts of nitrogen fertilizers strip the soil of beneficial minerals, resulting in the food with fewer minerals and vitamins.

On the other hand, organic cereals are grown under conditions where neither pesticides nor petrochemicals are allowed. Even after harvesting, nothing is introduced into the food supply: no fumigants, no rodenticides. In organic agriculture, the health of the soil is emphasized, which is why organic foods cost more.

On an organic farm, crops are rotated, and cover crops are used, which helps the soil to retain its carbon and nitrogen. Farmers avoid the use of pesticides by growing plants beside one another that naturally repel bugs. Fumigants and petrochemicals are prohibited. Sewage sludge, used as fertilizer on many conventional farms, may contain harmful contaminants such as asbestos and heavy metals and is banned at organic farms. By choosing "organic," we choose foods that still retain all their nutrients.

We also avoid pesticide residue, which becomes incorporated into the structure of conventionally grown foods and cannot be washed off. Lastly, when you choose organic, the food is neither bio-engineered (GM) nor irradiated.

TIME FOR A COMMERCIAL BREAK

"And when my doctor told me to increase my fiber, I decided to eat (Start My Day) every morning, cereal enriched with eight essential vitamins." How many TV ads have you listened to that describe a cereal *enriched* with essential vitamins? Few of us realize what that word, "enriched" really means. It means that the nutrients were removed during some stage of processing; In the case of flour, it's bleached to turn it white; with rice it is soaked and polished. Then because it lost most of its nutrients during the processing, laboratory-made vitamins need to be added in at the end.

What happened to the fiber that keeps things moving; the ones in those grains? Gone. And the antioxidants; all those super-nutrients like Vitamin E? Discarded, thrown into the rubbish, or have ended up at the end of a long drainage tube to feed the wastewater system. Do you see a problem here?

A TOUR INSIDE THE GRAIN

When we purchase a cereal made of whole grain, it is food resembling its natural state-closer to the soil it was grown in, rather than bleached and artificially colored. By choosing unprocessed grains, we enjoy food full of its original nutrients, the way nature intended. Each grain of a whole or stone-ground cereal contains three important parts. First, it wears a protective coat, called the *bran* to keep it safe from the elements. Some of us are familiar with bland bran cereals that taste like a cardboard box. I watched my grandmother eat them every day to motivate the contents of her intestine to start the rhumba. Can you believe this portion, which contains many nutrients was fed to chickens, pigs, and goats on farms, instead of being saved for the people? Those lucky little chicks were receiving all of the B vitamins and zinc needed by our immune systems. Perhaps that is why we never hear of chickens suffering from chronic fatigue. Whole grains also take longer to digest so they provide that satisfying fullness and stabilize blood sugar much better than grains, which are polished and bleached.

Beneath the bran is the endosperm. Sorry, it does not have anything to do with baby-making, though it sounds like it should. It is also full of nutrients, complex carbohydrates (carbs), and protein.

The innermost portion of the seed is called "the germ." This part is loaded with Enzymes; substances that speed up or slow down chemical reactions in our bodies. To create energy, digest food, or move a muscle, we need these chemical reactions. The 'germ' also contains fats, minerals, proteins, and vitamins. Maybe you have seen jars of Wheat Germ in your supermarket in the cereal aisle. People who eat this by spreading it on their morning cereal claim they have more energy.

When we eat whole grain cereals, we obtain the fiber everyone needs. When you are in your 20's, you may be able to get away with a diet full of French fries, pizza, and barely any vegetables or fruits. However, eating this way will get back at you in another ten years as our intestines need the roughage. Also, we need fiber in pretty high quantity. Did you know a person eating 2000 Calories a day needs at least 28 grams of fiber? Can you guess what the average American eats?

Usually 7 grams. No wonder we are bludgeoned with TV/internet ads for laxatives and stool softeners. Those ads are not just for retirees. The offices of GI doctors are flooded with men and women in their 30's and even with children, and many times, it is due to the food choices we make.

In order to explain this, I need to use some medical lingo. *Insoluble fiber*, one kind, is found in whole wheat, brown rice, whole grain corn, quinoa, spelt, millet and amaranth, which increases bulk, naturally drawing water into the stool to soften it. Now I sound like your doctor. This book may save you doctor and hospital visits when you can save your money by eating the right way.

To some people, organic cereals seem to lack the glamour that conventional cereals seem to offer. One thing they don't contain is high fructose corn syrup and may not taste as sweet at first. However, you can always add honey or some fresh or dried fruit, depending on the season, or add some nuts for added crunch.

I begin my day with organic Path Mesa Sunrise Cereal made of Indian corn, spelt, and amaranth, which gives me 6 grams of fiber and 4 grams of protein for every 3/4 cup serving. I sprinkle blueberries or dried cranberries over them. Sometimes I use a flavored milk such as vanilla, for variety. Another option is maple buckwheat flakes.

Because these are low-glycemic, meaning they will not raise the blood sugar excessively, they will keep you feeling full longer throughout the morning. These are rich in B vitamins and fiber, which reduce the chance of developing diabetes, obesity or diverticulosis. I also add a hard-boiled egg to the meal; the cereal and fruit does not contain enough protein to sustain me for the morning. Eggs can be hard-boiled the night before and kept refrigerated. Then all you need to do is, remove the shell.

IN PRAISE OF OATMEAL

On cold mornings, I enjoy organic instant oatmeal. It tastes great and you won't miss the preservatives. I use my favorite cereal bowl, the one embossed with a giant sunflower, and add to it 1/2 cup of boiling water, mix and eat. The directions for use with a microwave are different. For those of you with CFIDS, please avoid using a microwave oven. You have an illness caused by radiation and should avoid as many sources of radiation as possible. A bowl of oats makes a tasty and satisfying choice for lowering cholesterol and triglycerides and satisfies me along with a hard- or soft-boiled egg. I like to spoon applesauce and nuts over the oats. The apples are naturally high in pectin, another type of fiber, *soluble fiber* which our bodies need in order to produce short-chain fatty acids in the large intestine or colon, which bind to toxins inside the colon to be excreted. The walnuts provide protection from breast and prostate cancer. On days when I add raisins rather than applesauce, I am getting iron. All the time, I am getting the nutrients I need to fuel my body all morning. For those of you have more energy at night, you may enjoy preparing the recipes for Overnight oats, popular these days. As the name implies, you place the ingredients in the cup the night before. Tiny elves descend into your kitchen while you sleep, doing the work of turning this into something edible. The instant oatmeal is not the same as steel cut oats or old-fashioned oats but it is a step in the right direction. When you gain your energy, you can do the work of cooking oats with milk over the stove.

For a change of pace, cook up some quinoa flakes. This other hot cereal, closer in texture to cream of wheat, is light and fluffy and cooks in only 90 seconds. That's right, one and a half minutes! It doesn't provide the flavor that oatmeal will, so I need to be the kitchen maestro here, adding nuts, raisins, apple slices or dates to it. To my hot or cold cereals, I add a slice of whole grain toast for a more complete breakfast. Have you ever tasted the tart/sweet combo of orange marmalade? Dundees by Katies, made in the U.K. is a marmalade, free of corn syrup sweetener. I get an anti-oxidant boost having this spread. For those of you unfamiliar with it, marmalade is an orange jam that includes orange rind, where the nutrients lie. Those golden specks of orange peel are full of flavonoids, including *tangeritin* and *quercetin* found in several studies to prevent many cancers, including gastric, colorectal, lung, prostate, T-cell leukemia, lymph node metastasis, melanoma, breast cancer and leukemia HL-60.[10]

ADD A PIECE OF FRUIT TO COMPLETE

I choose fruit that doesn't require peeling to eat with my meals. There are plenty out there; organic pears and peaches, organic grapes as well as choices such as sliced, sweet juicy melon cut at the supermarket for you. For a sweet beverage, I choose 8 ounces of coconut water punched up with 4 ounces of anti-oxidant-rich pomegranate or black currant juice or I down a glass of tomato-based vegetable juice with its savory flavor. There are so many choices besides OJ. If you enjoy orange juice in the morning, buy the calcium-rich type to start your day with a good source of

---

[10] Zunli, Ke, Yu pan, Xiodan, Xu, Chao, Nie and Zhiqin, Zhou *Citrus* flavonoids and Human Cancers. *Journal of Food and Nutrition Research.* 2015; 3(5): 341-357. doi: 10.12691/JFNR-3-5-9

calcium and vitamin C. Many OJ's, even the organic type, now contain added vitamin D3, the sunshine vitamin, called that because sunshine is vital for our bodies to produce vitamin D. Research on flavonoids in OJ support the ideas these may provide protections against human breast and colorectal cancers.[11]

YES, YOU CAN EAT WAFFLES!

Are you stuck in the cold cereal zone? Escape from the boring routine by choosing organic frozen waffles & pancakes, both free of preservatives. It's way more fun to start the day eating the nubby grains of whole wheat waffles. Some come with the omega 3 oils from nutty-tasting flax or chia seeds in them. Explore those made with brown rice flour. Van's even makes gluten-free chocolate chip waffles for special occasions!

I toast whole grain pancakes and sandwich almond butter or sunflower seed butter in between them. Why did I not mention Peanut butter? Unless you are buying the unprocessed variety, peanut butter tends to be high in sugar. Top your waffles with fresh berries. I rarely use syrup on my pancakes and waffles, as it is too high on the glycemic scale. Yet I still enjoy sweet, enjoyable meals. I add a few slices of sunny mangoes from a jar in place of syrup, drizzling the juice along with them. Or I dollop

Greek vanilla yogurt with a scattering of strawberries on top. This breakfast provides me with antioxidants; calcium for my bones; and the staying power I need. I also receive the benefits of the good bacteria or probiotics found in the yogurt!

---

[11] Jaganathan, SK., Vellayappan, M.V., Narasimhan, G., & Supriyanto, E. Role of pomegranate and citrus fruit juices in colon cancer prevention. *World Journal of Gastroenterology* 2014 Apr 28; 20(16): 4618-4625.

INTRODUCING MILLET

Only 1/16 of an inch in size, this tiny grain, which grows as tall as stalks of corn, is high in protein. It repairs tissues and is loaded with the full miracle of that muscle-relaxing mineral, magnesium which I emphasize greatly in this health-boosting book.

Millet is one hardy grain, able to grow in places of drought where no other grain can survive, and it dates back to the Stone Age! If you read the Bible, you may have even noticed millet is mentioned to make bread!

This wonder grain is easy on the stomach. Bland tasting millet takes on the flavor of whatever you cook it in—tomato sauce, chicken broth, milk, or juice, making it most versatile. Enjoyed worldwide in places like Greece, Italy, China, India, and in Sudan—millet is widely popular outside the States. With so many people now gluten-sensitive, you will see millet in some breads and pasta at select stores.

I love having millet as a hot morning cereal, cooked in juice or milk, or enjoyed as a pilaf.

To 1/2 cup of uncooked millet, I add four parts (2 cups) of chicken broth seasoned with my favorite chicken soup spices, which for me are sage, rosemary, and thyme. I allow it to do its thing on the stove while I check Facebook or get the laundry done.

For those of you exhausted after a day of work and likely to fall over waiting for a meal to cook, I've provided a *-symbol in my meal plan section to indicate the grain needs to be cooked in advance for the next day's meal. The purpose of this is for you remember to cook it the night before, maybe while watching your favorite TV show.

QUINOA (KEEN-WAH)

Most grains cannot boast of being sources of protein but quinoa can! This grain that originated from the Incan civilization is easy to cook needing only a two to one ratio of fluid to the grain. And it is easy to digest! Quinoa is also a gluten-free grain providing 6 grams of fiber in each serving.

This tiny seed grain (commonly yellow but found in other colors such as red, pink, even black) grows under conditions similar to millet that other grains would not tolerate, such as drought. Growing on a stalk between 3 to 9 feet in height, the quinoa plant is considered a pseudo-grain, more closely related to spinach and beets. With its bitter saponin covering, which we wash off under running water, birds and insects are deterred from eating the quinoa. I use a fine sieve to rinse them. As the grains are so tiny, they're apt to fall through the holes of a conventional colander.

For centuries, the people of Ecuador, Chile, and Bolivia have enjoyed eating this light and fluffy grain. Three-thousand years ago, the Incas believed that quinoa was sent to them by their gods and enhanced their spirituality as well as endurance. I can see why they would associate it with endurance as quinoa is loaded with nutrients that provide energy; the B vitamin, riboflavin, which produces energy at the cellular level; folate, found in our red blood cells; manganese, which helps tissue to repair and protects the energy production factory, the mitochondria, from damage by free rads; and of course, magnesium, a co-factor in energy pathways. No wonder the ancients associated quinoa with good health! For the waist-watchers reading this, the grain is also low in fat and contains protective factors known as *lignans*, a nutrient also found in whole wheat, that wards off heart disease, breast cancer, and other cancers.

For people with damaged mitochondria, especially those diagnosed with SEID and CFIDS, this is super important. Here is a food that you want to incorporate into your life as much as possible. Why not start your day with a bowl of hot quinoa flakes that cook in only a minute and a half? I like to combine them in the bowl with a tablespoon of protein-rich, almond butter for even more staying power.

Quinoa breads are starting to appear on some store shelves as this book goes to press, and those with more energy may enjoy baking muffins with quinoa flour combined with leavening agents. Since quinoa lacks the elastic properties of wheat and won't rise, you will need to add a leavening agent such as *xanthan gum* when you bake with it. I store this white powder in my freezer because only a tiny amount is used at a time. I add it with my dry ingredients and it provides that stretchy texture to my breads and rolls.

For lunch, enjoy a quinoa pilaf, the cooked grain combined with your favorite veggies.

Supermarkets sell quinoa tabbouleh with veggies, commonly cucumber or bell peppers, or fruit such as raisins or cranberries. To plain quinoa, I add cucumbers, raw carrots, and red onions. (I like colorful meals), along with a light balsamic vinegar dressing. Whole Foods sells quinoa patties in the Deli area.

When Suppertime rolls around, you can serve quinoa pasta with a nutty pesto sauce alongside a hefty bowl of field greens. I can almost guarantee that when you start substituting quinoa in place of sandwiches, you will feel the difference; Better focus, and improved concentration. You can cook your quinoa one day, then refrigerate, and on a day when you eat soup, add 1/2 cup of the cooked quinoa to raise your protein and energy quotient. Useful in so many dishes: soups, salads, pilafs, tabbouleh, pasta, and breakfast cereals, quinoa provides a new world of dishes to enjoy!

RICE

One of the first foods we introduce to our babies, rice, feeds over two-thirds of the world's population. Its long history begins around 2500 B.C. in China with the grain's popularity growing to other parts of Asia, India, and the Mediterranean. Rice can be grown on every continent in the world except Antarctica! It requires moisture to grow this 3- to 5-foot-tall plant with its long slender leaves.

This grain is naturally gluten-free and low in fat. Mainly a carbohydrate food, rice contains a small amount of protein. Because it is not a complete protein, we eat it with foods that complement it, such as beans, soy products such as tofu, or cheese.

Rice is incorporated into many kinds of foods, including the Japanese wine, Sake, puddings, casseroles, pilafs, and breads and it comes in over 60 different varieties! Have you ever tried purple or black rice? These colored varieties boast more health-boosting nutrients than the white or brown variety. Although white and brown rice looks and tastes different; they are the same grain; The only difference is that white rice has had the husks removed. In order to make it white, it is polished, bleached, and further refined, removing much of its nutrient value.

Rice needs to be cooked with two to three times its volume of water, which softens the grain. As it absorbs the water, it inflates in the process. The rice you enjoy may be entirely different from the rice your neighbors around the block use. Diverse cultures employ different ways of cooking rice. Asians enjoy rice that sticks together, while rice served in an American restaurant is fluffy. An Italian restaurant would feature a risotto, with its creamy texture. Have fun deciding what ways rice works for you and your family.

An important grain to consume for those of us with chronic illness; you'll receive more benefits coming from brown rice, than white. By now, you may have heard that all rice, even organic, is contaminated with tiny amounts of arsenic. There is not much we can do to purchase rice free of this carcinogen. But since brown rice has not been bleached and rinsed in production the way white rice has, I advise soaking the rice the night before and then using extra water when cooking it to dilute the arsenic. Rice doesn't need to be boring! Are you familiar with Jasmine rice available as brown long-grain rice? This one is pleasantly aromatic and smells like popcorn as it cooks.

As with other grains, for years, it was mistakenly believed that the benefits of the grains reside in the endosperm or the germ, but new studies confirm that the good stuff resides in the *bran* layer, the part the farmers fed the animals with or threw away entirely. Bran besides motivating sluggish intestines, contains essential fats that can prevent inflammation in our bodies. What's that? PREVENTS INFLAMMATION? I woke some of my readers up with that one.

BROWN RICE FOR A SLENDER MIDDLE AND MORE

Polished white rice has lost many nutrients. When rice is milled or polished, between 67% to 80% of the vitamins and nutrients are nixed. Studies of people eating more whole grains and fewer refined ones, discovered people were less likely to gain weight than those eating refined grains such as white rice.[12]

---

[12] McKeown, N.M., Meigs, J.B.,Liu, S., Wilson, P.W.,& Jacques, P.F. (2002). Whole-grain intake is favorably associated with metabolic risk factors for type 2 diabetes and cardiovascular diseases in the Framingham Offspring Study. *American Journal of clinical nutrition,* 76(2). 390-398
https://doi.org/10/1093/ajcn/762.390

The benefits of rice don't stop with weight control, as a nutrient in it called *gamma-oryzanol*, has the ability to lower blood sugar. When blood sugar runs too high, you are diagnosed with Diabetes. So, we want to keep this number low. Where is this nutrient found? In the bran, of course. Two minerals—magnesium (which acts as a co-factor in our ability to regulate both glucose and insulin) and manganese (which makes up an enzyme used in energy production inside our mitochondria) are found in brown rice. Have I yet convinced you to eat brown rice? Another mineral, selenium, found in rice, is involved in many metabolic pathways, especially those of our thyroid gland, that hidden gland found inside the front of our neck. The butterfly-shaped thyroid gland secretes hormones that regulate our weight, body temperature, and heart rate. Hormones are held in check better in those eating brown rice because whole grains, such as brown rice, whisk the toxins out of our body, improving the hormone profile. Selenium also partners up with vitamins A and C as part of our immune system, to scavenge free radicals.

What's even more important news about rice and selenium is that this mineral works with *glutathione* (that sure is a mouthful, huh?) Glutathione is a nutrient found in our livers that breaks down the toxic stuff our bodies come into contact with. People with SEID ad CFIDS are found to have lower glutathione levels than normal and need to receive supplemental glutathione or take NAC, which is a precursor to this nutrient. A most important body part, our livers have so many fascinating functions to keep our bodies running! We also want our brains and nervous systems to be at their best; we need the choline, which makes up brain and spinal cord matter found in brown rice; vitamin E (which recycles vitamin C in our bodies); folic acid, essential for the development of the neural tube in utero; and three other B vitamins. Finally, people eating whole grain brown rice have fewer blood clots making them less prone to dangerous embolisms, strokes, and heart attacks.

CHAPTER 4

SNACKS

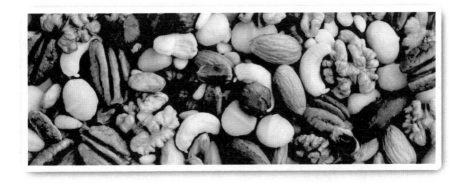

KEEP HUNGER PANGS AT BAY WITH SMART SNACKS

Have you ever fallen asleep on your dinner plate? I have. My mother once said, "Well Mary, if you are that tired, why don't you just go to bed? "After wiping the mashed potato off my face, I must have sleep-walked my way back up to my room on the third floor. Sometimes sleep is more important. So take that rest, and then eat a healthy snack when you wake up. If you wake in the morning, with hardly any appetite, save the fruit from your planned breakfast to eat later with *hummus* or a stick of cheese, two great protein choices. Hummus, a tasty mixture of chickpeas with tahini, is available in several varieties with the addition of red peppers, olives, artichokes, or garlic. I like to grill a corn tortilla or toast a gluten-free pita and then spread the hummus on it.

To keep our blood sugar steady, we need to eat healthy snacks often. When blood sugar sags, we lag. Even our brain cells will be slowed, making it hard to concentrate and feel your best when your blood sugar is tanking. These days a new word has been coined, Hangry. No this is not a mis-print. Hangry is a real condition identified in 2017, describing people who are very hungry experiencing anger. Do you find yourself blowing up at your colleagues just before lunch? Are you the victim of someone else's Hanger? Perhaps someone's road rage? The solution can be as simple as eating more often to keep the blood sugar stable. So maybe you want to grab some cheese sticks or a protein-rich smoothie for that "monster" in your office, or maybe he/she resides in your home.

Research in multiple studies bears out that skipping meals, especially Breakfast, leads to negative outcomes on our cardiovascular health. According to a review of multiple studies published in the respected medical journal, *Circulation*, "Greater eating frequency is associated with a lower LDL cholesterol," the unfavorable portion of cholesterol that we want to lower! Eating frequent meals is also associated with a lower risk of obesity.[13] These

---

[13] St.-Onge, MP., Ard, J., Buskin, M.L., Chiuve, S.E., Johnson H.M., Etherton, P.K., and Varady, K. Meal Timing and Frequency: Implications for Cardiovascular Disease Prevention: A Scientific Statement from the American Heart Association. *Circulation*

studies were so strong that the American Heart Association created a Position Statement on the importance of eating frequent meals. Eating more often is going to prevent "hanger" but also will keep the blood sugar steady so that you don't build up that giant "I-can-eat-everything-in-the-house" appetite. Nevertheless, it's the content of the snacks that matters, especially when you take medications with a side effect of lowering blood sugar. (Many of the NSAIDS do). Eating a handful of crackers provides a small amount of energy and, in some of us, could induce a blood sugar spike, followed by a crash but combining the crackers with some cheese, a protein food, decreases drowsiness and fatigue that a snack of crackers alone (pure carbs) creates.

I am super aware of the presence of hormones and antibiotics in my food, and you should be too. Germs resistant to most antibiotics such as the flesh-eating bacteria, M.R.S.A and the stomach-upsetting, E. Coli infection, are more prevalent due to antibiotics fed to chickens and cows on conventional farms.

To avoid hormone and antibiotic residue, assure you are really eating 100% cheese, by choosing organic or imported cheese. Horizon Organics sells individually-wrapped mozzarella and Colby Jack cheese sticks to slip inside a pocket or purse.

I enjoy imported Provolone cheese with its sharp bite, free of both of these. I grew up on this cheese, with my Italian Nana feeding this to us frequently. Bring along an apple or pear or carry a small plastic bag filled with grapes or raisins to eat with the cheese. Keep a canister of dried plums, aka, "prunes," in a nearby cabinet or the drawer of your desk to eat with a protein snack, (Greek yogurt, peanut butter, or cheese). Greek yogurt is a real hit in this country. With a texture similar to cheesecake, it is a most satisfying yogurt providing 9 grams of protein. You can always add granola or fruit to add extra flavor and crunch.

If you've had a bad day, what are you likely to turn to? Most of us tear into a package of cookies or candy to soothe frazzled nerves. Did you know this knee-jerk reaction of turning to comfort food began early in life? When we had a total meltdown in aisle 3, or we were crying after a shot from the pediatrician, Mom might have calmed us down with a cookie; thus, we've come to view sweet snacks as "comfort foods." Snacking can also be a useful way to attain nutrients that meals by themselves may not supply. For example, after a large meal, I am usually too full to eat an orange as dessert. I know by 8 p.m., though, while watching TV, hunger returns, and I'm searching for something to eat. When I walk into the kitchen to check that the house- elves have not magically scrubbed my dirty dishes sitting in the sink, that juicy orange I purposely left out on the counter, greets me. Anyone who has ever followed a diet realizes that "Out of sight is out of mind," so if it isn't in full view, I tend to forget it even exists. If you are forgetful, (and this is very common with long-haulers), you may want to have some post-it notes handy in the kitchen. I write little notes that I stick on my fridge to remember some foods do require refrigeration.

When you choose any snack, be sure to read the ingredient label. If you see the words, *hydrogenated* or *partially hydrogenated*, seen often on the labels of peanut butter, and on some loaves of bread, you will know that artery-clogging trans fats are added to the food. Fortunately, many hydrogenated fats have been removed from products, but some still linger. Because staying away from trans fats is so important to us all, you will frequently see these words mentioned in this book. You also want to look for grams of fiber on the label. Fiber, which was discussed in Chapter 3, is important for many reasons. However, did you know Fiber itself supplies nutrients?

PROTEIN POWER FOODS

Take a walk down the Peanut butter aisle at your supermarket. Take notice that it's not only peanut butter that's being sold. Next to it are jars of almond butter, cashew butter, soy butter, and sunseed butter, to name a few. All are high in protein, providing 4 grams of energy to sustain you through that traffic nightmare on the way home or to get you through that meeting with your dissertation advisor. Nuts, as well as seeds are also loaded with vitamin E and a multitude of minerals. All of our metabolic systems need minerals to function, many working as co-factors in reactions to create energy out of the food we eat. For a high protein snack, spread nut and seed butters on whole rye crackers or gluten free Breton crackers.

MMMMM, YOGURT!

Many supermarkets now display yogurt parfaits sold near or in the produce department. While they are a healthier snack than a candy bar, these yummy snacks full of berries and granola may offer a bit more sugar than you want. Have you noticed some yogurts have 22 grams of sugar in them? Beware if the first ingredient listed is sugar!! Between the chocolate chips and the peanut butter chips, they are practically candy! Why not make your own parfaits? I make eating yogurt something to look forward to by layering a swath of creamy vanilla yogurt with crunchy flakes of Muesli or adding the midnight blue of berries to my lemon yogurt. This not only looks great, but the anthocyanin in both blueberries and blackberries enhance memory and benefit our eyes. Tempting your tastebuds with foods that look attractive will seduce your appetite when you lack the energy to eat. Suppose you are not able to tolerate yogurt from a cow. In that case, there are plenty of options available, including kefir-based, made from goats' milk, almond milk, coconut milk yogurts, cashew milk, rice milk, and even soy milk, which was the original non-dairy yogurt. *SO* the brand makes delicious coconut milk-based yogurts such as peach, Key lime pie, pineapple Brulee, and spiced blueberry. If purchasing the soy variety, always choose organic. Soy is one of those crops that receives tons of pesticides in the form of genetically engineering. By buying organic, you don't need to worry about these possibly harmful practices. You will enjoy *The Stonyfield* line of dairy-free organic soy yogurts, featuring, raspberry, blueberry, and vanilla-raspberry, or try *Nancy's Creamy* strawberry soy yogurt or Raspberry soy yogurt.

Have you ever wondered why yogurt is so popular? It is a cultured milk product, originally made from cows' milk. The bacterial cultures used in making yogurt are probiotics that populate our gut. They are probiotics and do the exact opposite that antibiotics do. While antibiotics, which means "against life," are designed to KILL organisms, a probiotic "pro" meaning "for life," promotes the healthy viability of bacteria in our intestine, which we need for our immune system. Again, choose organic when you buy the cows' milk form, because you do not want the antibiotic and hormone residue routinely used on conventional factory farms.

For the adventurous among us, kefir made from goat's milk with its strong tang may be a refreshing snack or a dessert. For those unfamiliar with kefir, it is a cultured milk drink but made from goat's milk rather than cow's milk and provides the same bacterial strains. I enjoy the mango and the strawberry. You can also buy frozen kefir which is like eating ice cream. For those allergic to cow's milk, kefir makes a nice alternative. You will read more about dairy snacks like yogurt and kefir in later chapters.

NUTS!

A handful of potassium-rich nuts becomes a satisfying and crunchy snack with numerous benefits, including lowering cholesterol's unfavorable LDL. Even though this protein-rich food is high in fat, nuts boast the best kind; the mono-unsaturated - good for the heart kind. Nuts contain more goodies; potassium, an important electrolyte which our bodies need for all our muscles, especially our hearts! Did you know potassium is one of those magic minerals that lowers blood pressure and keeps it from rising too high? Almonds-unsalted, rich in calcium, contain over 700 mg. of potassium. Hazel nuts follow along the potassium continuum with 680 mg. Cashews and Brazil nuts tie with 659 mg of potassium. And then there are Brazil nuts, which help blue moods to take a hike. In addition, you don't need to eat a handful of them to gain this benefit in mood. Just one Brazil nut a day does the trick. Of course, if you take prescription anti-depressants, you don't want to ditch your meds without talking to your doctor. Nuts are an admirable Vitamin E source, which recycles vitamin C. Moreover, for those who are concerned about intestinal traffic jams, nuts are fiber-rich gems that keep moving things smoothly through the GI tract. Just be sure and chew them really well.

If you want your nuts to last longer, store them in the freezer and place in an air tight container for up to 4 months at a time. Now you may be aware of new information about *acrylamide.* This carcinogen is found in foods that are roasted or baked to a brown color. Roasted nuts are in this category, unfortunately. If this concerns you, then buy raw nuts and soak them. I really enjoy the flavor of roasted nuts, so I'm not sure I can take this step.

SEEDS AND STUFF

Similar in nutrients to nuts are seeds like: pumpkin, sesame, and sunflower, and chia. I often grab a handful of zinc-rich pumpkin seeds for a snack. These powerful immune boosters contain both potassium and vitamin E. Chew them well before swallowing— especially if you have been diagnosed with *diverticulosis*, a condition where the intestines form small pouches or pockets easily irritated by undigested seeds and nuts.

Smooth green pumpkin seeds, loaded with Zinc, the immune-boosting mineral, are a great addition to yogurt or ice cream or enjoyed by themselves. All seeds are rich in fiber, which increases movement in our GI tract. How many of you enjoy snacking on sunflower seeds? These zebra-striped nuggets are rich in vitamin E and the same type of mono-unsaturated fat as nuts. Any combination of seeds, fruit, and nuts can be used to make a trail mix. As long as you don't see the word, *hydrogenated* or *partially hydrogenated* on the ingredient label, you are buying a healthy package of seeds. Go ahead! Sprinkle them on ice cream, pair them with yogurt, scatter black sesame seeds over your salads and cream cheese, add them to hot and cold cereals or sneak some into to your home-baked cookies and your cooked grain dishes such as quinoa and rice.

PROTEIN + CARBS = LASTING ENERGY

When you snack smartly, you combine foods found in the protein group with food from the carbohydrate group. We pair protein foods without even thinking about it because they taste good together. Think cheese and crackers, peanut butter and crackers, hummus and raw veggies, yogurt and granola. By combining the proteins with the carbs rather than just eating carbs by themselves.

we fuel our bodies with high-octane fuel for more endurance and better mileage. In addition, we prevent hypoglycemia by keeping the blood sugar on an even keel. The chart below gives you examples of protein and carbohydrate foods you can pair. Choose one food from the left column and one from the right, and you are good to go!

SNACK COMBOS

Protein Foods	Carbohydrate Foods
cheese	crackers, bread, fruit
nuts, seeds	ice cream, cereal
hummus	crackers, bread, celery, carrots
hardboiled eggs	breads, biscuits, crackers
yogurt	raisins, dried plums, granola, crackers
deli turkey breast	lettuce leaf, crackers, bread, rice
cup of bean soup	crackers, leftover grain such as rice, millet, small salad
peanut butter and other nut butters	rice cakes, crackers, crisp breads, bread

Some of you may have concluded that there isn't a big difference between a snack and a meal. They are reversible, and you can be as flexible as you desire. There's no rule that bans having a bowl of oatmeal with some fruit as your dinner! Even some restaurants make breakfast options available day and night. If you work from home, you don't need to do the same degree of planning as those running out the door in the morning to get to work. You also have the freedom to snack throughout the day.

You might choose a soup and salad from the chart for a meal and become too fatigued to eat the salad after heating the soup. Simply save it in a clear container in the fridge or bring it with you into the room you will be in, and have a bite now and then.

Have you ever wondered about what happens to the foods we eat? How exactly do the foods on your plate become processed into energy? Let's take a journey through our digestive tract to see how the system actually works.

WELCOME TO YOUR DIGESTIVE TRACT

You may need to bring a flashlight - it's so dark in here with many winding paths. We're inside the mouth, where the chocolate caramel turtle is welcomed. Even though it seems as though that pecan goodie gets glued directly onto your left hip, it actually doesn't work that way. The master plan is to ship food along the digestive canal, leading to the stomach's industrial area, and where strong acids are created to dissolve food materials. These are then sent out through sophisticated tubing we call our intestines for processing. What cannot be processed is considered waste and is excreted at the end of the line. The stomach breaks foods down into nutrients we can use but needs other organs to help in the process of refining nutrients. Our liver, gall bladder, and pancreas are all in on the action. There are still some tickets left to visit these places. Along the journey, from entry to exit via the rectum, things can go wrong. It's like arriving at an airport in Milan at 2 p.m., but your luggage traveled on to Hong Kong.

If the problems were strictly mechanical, digestion and absorption might occur with few glitches, but our GI tracts are super sensitive to stress. This is why our stomachs clench when we receive bad news; we get dry mouth when it's performance review time or feel nauseous waiting to see the lawyer. Our nervous system is highly intertwined with the GI tract and newer research bears out that our immune system is found along its borders. Anyone suffering from IBS, commonly known as *irritable bowel syndrome*, knows that when faced with a deadline or the constant battles with the ex-spouse, the colon delivers more and faster than intended, with that constant need to use the bathroom.

Let's return to the opposite end; where we started at the mouth. Inside, we find two tiers of living structures, our pearly whites, whose job is to grind up the animal and plant parts we eat for meals. Many of us don't even consider teeth as a living material, but they have a blood and nerve supply. As infants and children, our teeth grow rapidly. After adulthood, the growth slows down but still occurs. Remember the saying, "Long in the tooth" referring to really old Senior citizens? Our salivary glands secrete enzymes called *salivary amylase*, which begins the digestion of some foods right in the mouth. This is limited to carbohydrate foods. Both the enzymes and water secreted by our glands along the jawline, dilute and soften the food.

However, along with the teeth and the saliva is another structure inside our mouths that gets in on the action; the tongue. This pink paddle-shaped organ is covered in muscles and sensors on its surface called our taste buds, which makes eating a pleasure! Our tongues mechanically push food toward the next area, the throat, which opens into a long canal called the *esophagus*. Food is now on its journey to the stomach at the other end of this long tube.

As referred to previously, the stomach is a factory where very potent *hydrochloric acid* is pumped out, strong enough to burn a hole in a sofa cushion. This substance is used to break down Protein foods (steak, eggs, peanut butter, chicken) into their building blocks or peptides. Other digestive enzymes are available to dissolve food materials even further. The stomach also jostles things around to mechanically pulverize food materials; much like the agitator inside our washing machines.

The resultant mash next passes through a valve called the pyloric valve into a series of tubes we refer to as the small and large intestines. The small intestine does most of the work. It's analogous to a luxury summer resort with all its offerings residing in various locations. Horseback riding is offered in the north field, par 18 golf course in the east, and the water park in the sunny southwest. Each area has its own specialized function with a specially trained staff. More enzymes are produced here to break down proteins and fats. The pancreas sends over its *pancreatic amylase* enzyme and whatever is left of carbs (that cookie with the chocolate chunks).

A specific part of the small intestine is used for breaking down double sugars into simple sugars so they can be absorbed into the bloodstream. The protein foods, BBQ chicken leg, tofu loaf, filet mignon) breaks down into peptides in the stomach and now further degrade in the intestine to amino acids where they are carried to the liver, muscles, and other cells.

Carbs, such as the pears with maple syrup and those red bliss potatoes, all end up as glucose, which feeds our brain and muscles. The Fats (butter, French fries, guacamole) cannot be digested in the stomach, instead they reach the intestines ready to be dismantled by a hormone produced by the gall bladder. These are absorbed through the lining of the small intestine. Next, they are transferred to the liver or sit around in the blood stream as fatty acids. It's these fats that interest our primary care practitioners so much that they test as part of our annual physical. Your health care provider then calls you in to go over the report with you and tells you that your LDL is too high and your HDL is too low, from enjoying all those hamburgers, steaks and French fries.

Abutting the intestines, are immune system cells ready to pounce on anything that gets onto their side of the property line. Blood vessels surround the intestinal walls where normally only microscopic particles of food get through. However, certain conditions can damage the intestinal lining, allowing large particles of food to get through the walls. WATCH OUT! This could signal trouble in the form of developing food sensitivities, which I will go into detail about later in this book.

You see, the membrane lining the wall of the intestine is supposed to work in a particular way. The Great Creator designed it with a certain size pore to create an efficient means of absorbing totally digested nutrients, (amino acids from protein, glucose from carbs, fatty acids, and glycerol from fats). Then they can enter the bloodstream to travel where needed. For example, with their nitrogen groups, amino acids enter a construction zone where proteins are built into tissues such as muscle. Those of us unable to exercise have a nasty process happen to our muscles; atrophy or withering from not being used. Another reason doctors emphasize the importance of exercise.

Whether from toxin exposure or pollution or from eating foods laced with preservatives, some people develop pores in the intestinal membrane that are too large and allow undigested food particles to escape into the bloodstream. The results can be nausea, gas, headaches, fatigue, bloating, and achy joints as the immune system reacts to mount a defense. The immune cells located all along the intestinal wall send out antibodies, usually to our favorite foods, the ones you feel you simply would perish without-such as bread. In Chapter 10, you will learn about food intolerances and how they can be treated.

In the next chapter, I will share some simple meal planning strategies with you to upgrade your favorite meals boosting their nutrition content without a whole lot of extra work. Who says "lunch' foods cannot be eaten as dinner or 'breakfast' foods cannot be enjoyed at noon? The food police are not going to raid your house at 6 p.m. to see what foods are on your dinner table. I combine protein-rich eggs with vegetables at any time of day, such as creating a meal around a salad with hard boiled eggs or combining eggs with a frozen fish fillet on a bed of curly green lettuce and adding my favorite veggies. Other days I combine eggs with the already cooked greens sitting in my fridge and add some dried onion, shredded cheese, and my favorite salad dressing. It's easy. On more energetic days, I make an omelet or frittata with eggs and vegetables.

CHAPTER 5

INTERCHANGEABLE MEALS

E ven the old PB and J of our childhoods can be upgraded to a sandwich with more lasting power. Let's replace white bread with whole-grain sprouted wheat bread, use fruit preserves instead of sugary jam, and choose natural peanut butter to reduce the sugar content while boosting the antioxidants.

Old PB & J made with white bread and jelly	New PB & J made with whole grain bread and unsweetened jam
0 grams of fiber	3 grams of fiber in the bread
32-36 grams of sugar	10 grams of sugar
may contain high fructose corn syrup in jelly and peanut butter	preserves are made with cane sugar and pectin to thicken. Natural peanut butter is 100% peanuts, no sugar added.
147 mg of sodium	120 mg. of sodium

Your peanut butter and jam sandwich made this way is full of the B vitamins: thiamin, vitamin B6 (important for our nerves), riboflavin—an energy vitamin, and magnesium. Since riboflavin, also found in milk, is full of energy potential, it makes sense for us to load up on riboflavin-rich foods like nut butters and enjoy that glass of cold milk with the sandwich!

Peanut butter being a high protein food contains 2 valuable minerals; zinc and iron. By switching out the strawberry jam for lower sugar strawberry preserves, you give your immune system a boost. Feeling adventurous? Switch out the strawberry with other berry spreads such as blackberry, elderberry, or raspberry. How many other all-fruit spreads can you find at your farmer's market or supermarket?

You just returned from the blood lab where the tech could not overcome her vampire tendencies and extracted 5 tubes of blood from your vein. Now you feel drained.

Blood draws are particularly exhausting for those of us with a lowered blood volume, a condition often found in those with fibromyalgia and/or CFIDS. Are you now too exhausted to cook? Or even to eat? Does this feeling of bone-weary, collapsing- 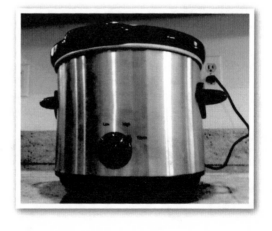 to-the-floor exhaustion persist for another two or three days? Then, it's time to enlist the aid of a helper to do your cooking for you. If no chef is available on the premises to pamper you, you can always rely on a slow cooker, or crockpot, that will have a wholesome meal ready at home when you walk through the door at the end of the day. I know the microwave is faster, but we want to eliminate as many sources of radiation in our food as possible to become well! We want nutrients from our foods in top form.

Stalwart stews and comforting casseroles, even a roasted chicken, can be made in the slow cooker. The secret of the slow cooker is food cooks in a great deal of fluid and at a much lower temperature than on the stove so that you can rest in bed or lie on the couch until the incredible aroma beckons you into the kitchen to eat. You can make a meal using precut chunks of veal, chicken, beef, or pork or you can as well keep it vegetarian with an assortment of legumes and colorful vegetables.

Now for news some of you may not like: You can't eat red meat every single day. It's not good to have that much in your system. In fact, we all need to put the brakes on our consumption of red meat, limiting it to one or two serving per week. Why? Way back in 2008, the National Institute of Health (NIH), changed the guidelines for meat consumption in this country to a maximum of two servings of red meat per week. If you still need your red meat fix, choose grass-fed which supplies more of the nutrients that we need and less of the saturated fat than meat from Feed-lot cattle fed conventionally. Grass-fed supplies us with more nutrients, which our bodies require. Remember, we are building a higher nutrient to junk ratio. We receive a higher amount of CLA or *conjugated linoleic acid* in the meat from the grass-fed cows—and it tastes better! CLA has been found to increase metabolism and assists in weight reduction.[14] Who doesn't want a more efficient metabolism?

---

[14] Kennedy, A., Martinez, K., Schmidt, S., Mandrup, S., LaPoint, K., & McIntosh, M. Antiobesity mechanisms of actions of conjugated linoleic acid. *The Journal of Nutritional Biochemistry*, 21(3), 171-179 https://doi.org/10.1016/j.jnutbio.2009.08.003

And I know many of you want to lose weight! Now you probably wonder about the taste. It is simply delicious!

In 2010, information was released that all American beef except organic, has become contaminated with copper, pesticides, and antibiotic residue, which can lead to kidney failure. This can become very serious and lead to death. Now I sound like an advertisement for a medication!

The poor quality of the conventional American beef came to light following a refusal by our Southern neighbor, Mexico, who refused to accept any American beef due to this contamination. Organic beef now boasts the B vitamins, thiamine, B12, folic acid, plus the mineral, iron. Free-range beef and poultry are preferable to those from conventional farms because the cattle eat grass, which is converted in their bodies to healthier muscle tissue, which is the steak, hamburger, and roasts we eat. Our feathered friends, walk around freely eating produce scraps and receive feed supplemented with omega 3 fatty acids. On conventional farms, cattle and chicken are rarely given this supplemental feed and are instead fed corn to fatten them quickly as well as the consumer who sits down to that chicken dinner.

When using a slow cooker, combine tough cuts of meat with any three or more of these: carrots, organic corn, chickpeas, green beans, organic celery, pinto beans, black-eyed peas, mushrooms, and potatoes, white, orange or yellow. These are sturdy vegetables that cook well over extended periods, whereas vegetables with higher water content, such as tomatoes or zucchini, will melt into the fluids. You can always add them later.

When you can barely make it up a flight of stairs, you don't have the energy to slice vegetables, so make it easy and buy frozen. You can purchase just about any vegetable in its frozen state. Most come already sliced or diced. Just add them to the slow cooker.

Some supermarkets sell pre-cut vegetables for stews such as turnips, parsnips, potatoes, and carrots in the produce aisle, making it easy to put a meal together.

THE IRON CLAD GUARANTEE

My grandmother owned a heavy cast-iron skillet that was never stored beneath the cabinets where the other pans were stored. No, this baby had the place of honor, right on top of the stove. Into its smoother interior would go the chicken cutlets she was frying on Tuesday nights. Tuesday night was always cutlet night (veal or chicken, depending on the economy). Out of that sleek skillet, the golden artichoke frittatas, fluffy Sunday-morning pancakes, and crispy strips of bacon would magically appear. Even when non-stick coatings were popular, Grandma stuck to her use of that enormous black cast-iron fry pan. Did you know that cast-iron cookware is making a comeback?

There are at least two good reasons:
1. This cookware actually enhances the iron content of the food cooked inside of it.
2. The thick layers of iron making up the pan spread heat evenly, so food is less likely to burn.

So instead of sticking your hamburger beneath the broiler to cook, you may want to invest in the use of a cast-iron pan instead.

CAUTION:

The alarm to alert the cooking police will be activated if you cook broccoli or cauliflower for long periods as the cooking process itself intensifies flavors, and the neighbor living above you will be attaching a clothespin to his nose, complaining about the stench.

Clean up can be just as easy as with a non-stick coated pan but is different. It would be best if you keep the iron pan "seasoned." Rather than washing it with soap and water, we wipe away food particles with a paper towel, then grease the inside with olive oil regularly and heat it on low heat to maintain a non-stick surface. The thick layers or iron spread heat evenly, so food is less likely to burn.

WARNING: Cast-iron pans weigh about 30 lbs. when empty. For those of us with weak neck and upper body muscles, hefting one of these could trigger pain that can last several days.

IRON-RICH MEALS YOU WILL SAVOR

Although we are limiting our beef consumption, we are not yet aiming for total sainthood, so here comes the night when we celebrate life with steak and peppers. The sautéed peppers add sweet flavor and are rich in immunity-boosting vitamin C—bell peppers, when cooked in the cast-iron pan, double the available iron content of the steak.

The good news is you don't need to sit down to a bag of nails to obtain all the iron your body needs. It wouldn't do any good anyway as iron needs to be in a digestible form. Lean beef, lamb, veal, and fish are the best sources of this mineral we need for our blood. We find it iron in our red blood cells as *heme* iron. Other iron rich foods referred to as *non-heme* iron include beets, peanuts, peanut butter, whole wheat bread, crackers, brown rice, and blackstrap molasses. For those unfamiliar with it, black strap molasses is my go-to when I serve baked beans. It is a sweet thick syrup and is a great source of iron. I relish adding this molasses, free of sulfur, to tea as well.

A meal featuring non-heme iron would be pasta and beans, an Italian entree enjoyed in many places. If a vegetarian, you probably enjoy adding tomato sauce to many of your bean dishes. I grew up eating pasta and beans or *Pasta Fagioli* although I did not enjoy it at that time. The size of the pasta used effects the quality of the dish. Tiny pasta, tubettini, for example, soaks up more of the fluid resulting in a pasty entree. Using large elbow macaroni allows more sauce to float over the pasta, making it lighter.

If you're vegetarian, you wouldn't think of not eating your greens. Your plate is commonly loaded with dark green leafies, a source of non-heme iron. Well, you can boost the amount of iron your body absorbs by having a glass of orange juice with the meal. I know that some have finicky stomachs that cannot tolerate OJ well, especially if you have a reflux condition. The supermarkets offer low acid varieties of OJ that may be more tolerable. Matty's organic OJ is sweeter and less likely to bother my stomach.

S-L-O-W-I-N-G DOWN:

Iron picks up a protein called *hemoglobin* found in our red blood cells, and this molecule carries oxygen to where it is needed. What else happens besides exhaustion when we are not receiving enough iron? Strangely enough, a blood test may fail to detect a deficiency during the early stages, but our brains will register the deficit. Difficulty in concentrating, memory problems, and having an attention span of a gnat, are common when you have a less than clinical iron deficiency. Do you have a miserable memory? For women, having menstrual periods puts us at risk for iron deficiency, especially if we have heavy blood loss. As iron deficiency continues, the skin becomes pale as the tissues are not being saturated with oxygen-rich blood and you may become sensitive to cold. Are you wearing three sweaters inside the house? Your heart may begin its own little dance. Well, at least one part of the body is exercising.

By the time you drag yourself into the doctor's office with all these symptoms, your health provider will most likely diagnose you with *anemia*. This means you liver stores of iron have dropped so much, putting you in danger if you don't receive treatment. Scientists know that anemia is linked to many infections and have lately linked anemia to weakening and disability in the elderly. Unfortunately, those with chronic fatigue syndrome, and CFIDS, and unable to exercise, suffer from many things that our parents and grandparents suffer from. Blood work from people with CFS shows the same degree of damage to older adults' oxygen pathways.[15] This actually reflects the loss of strength that many have in getting up from a chair. For some of us on certain days, it is major exertion!

---

[15] Fulle, S., Mecocci, P., Fano, G., Vecchiet, I. Vecchini, A., Racciotti, D., & Beal. M.F. (2000) Specific Alterations in vastus lateralis muscle of patients with the diagnosis of chronic fatigue syndrome. Free Radical Biology and Medicine, 29(12), 1252-1259.

10 MINUTE MEALS

You want to increase your energy, right? Isn't that why you picked up this book? I will guide you along the highway to improved health and energy. Building meals around grains is another route to high-energy meals. However, they need to be WHOLE ones. Earlier, you learned how to create meals starting with soup. Now it's time to include more fiber and B vitamins at every meal. If you have a few pounds to lose, the extra fiber is going to be your new BFF. If you are naturally slender, the fiber will still be beneficial. Let's start with Barley. With its nutty taste, this cereal grain is often used to thicken broths while also supplying us with fiber and selenium. Selenium is a mineral that makes up *glutathioine* to detoxify the things in our bodies we don't need.

A plain broth might leave you hungry, but a nice organic chicken or beef broth thickened with pearl barley is more nourishing and far more satisfying. Plus, you get the benefit of soluble fiber high in *beta glucans* which lowers cholesterol and blood sugar, plus its high in the B vitamins, folate and choline.

Barley is available in several forms - quick cooking, which has been steamed ahead of time and takes only 15 minutes to cook, and pearl, which takes longer to cook (45 minutes). Both are high in B vitamins and very filling. When I make chicken soup, I open a carton of organic chicken broth to which I add chunks of celery, carrots, and sprigs of parsley plus barley to thicken, creating a heartier meal. You can substitute barley in place of the pasta or rice you usually add for a change of pace. Barley does contain gluten, so those of you with Celiac disease or gluten sensitivity may not want to use it. You can add instant brown rice to the broth or millet that you cooked from a previous meal.

Are you familiar with *couscous?* This Moroccan pasta doesn't even need to cook. Similar to instant rice in its simplicity, the seed-like grain made of wheat is a bit fluffier than rice. You simply boil water in a pan and pour the couscous into the water, then remove it from the heat. It's that simple. It tastes divine with a sprinkle of my favorite herbs: mint, parsley, sage, or cooked in orange juice rather than water.

MEAL BUILDING TIME

Creating a meal is really like architecture for dummies. We know we need to have three foods in our diet: Protein, Fat, and Carbohydrate. We are using these basic tools to build meals by adding vegetables to our grains. Make it as colorful and adventurous as you want: Frozen snow peas, crunchy water chestnuts with a sprinkling of ground ginger, and snippets of scallions blended with some duck sauce. In the frozen food aisle, you'll find bags and boxes of Chinese vegetables, including broccoli, carrots, and snow peas. Look for the label that does not include a salty sauce loaded with preservatives and fattening corn syrup. They are so convenient without any need to defrost them. Just dunk them into boiling water without defrosting, then add some diced garlic and low sodium soy sauce along with a few green onions and garlic.

You may prefer to use the less pungent garlic powder if you are going to be around other people. Save the crushed garlic for those nights when you are staying home, alone.

GO MEXICAN!

Based on another grain, corn, we have Mexican and Spanish food: colorful, festive, sizzling hot and spicy, right? What comes to mind for many people is indigestion! However, Mexican food can be enjoyed without the fire of hot peppers. In fact, it can be quite mild when you make it yourself. Who doesn't enjoy a burrito, taco, or Mexican salad occasionally? You control the *calienté* and create a fun meal that the entire family will enjoy.

In a large skillet with enough water to cover the bottom, I brown a pound of lean ground turkey in place of ground beef. When it becomes dry, I just add a tablespoon of water at a time to the pan to prevent the contents from drying out and burning.

Then I drain the meat and dust it with chili powder or use a pre-made taco- seasoning packet without MSG or preservatives. You'll find them in the healthier food section of your supermarket, I add a can of red kidney beans for a fiber boost, which boasts close to 6 grams of fiber for every half cup. Canned beans don't require soaking overnight, but they do need to be rinsed and drained, then added to the meat.

Final touches are crispy leaves of romaine, slices of tomato, and pre-shredded Monterey jack cheese and corn kernels. Last, I add the piquant flavor of salsa—no longer limited to just the tomato kind. For a change of pace, try a sweet peach, mango or pineapple salsa.

Hunt down the corn tortillas or your taco shells. When getting a meal ready for the family, take the easy way out by placing each ingredient on a paper plate on the table. This way, each member assembles her food at the table, the way she likes. The kids will absolutely love this! There is only one pan to clean, the one you used to brown the meat.

When it comes to purchasing corn products such as taco shells, I opt for organic only, as most of the corn in this country is genetically modified. Even though manufacturers tell us that there is no difference in eating GM foods, I beg to differ. The incidence of irritable bowel disease is growing exponentially. Do you ever consider it could be from the genetic manipulation of our food supply? Corn and Soy are not even desired by other countries when it comes to t rade which has nothing to do with tariffs. Genetically modified corn contains something called *glyphosate*, which is a pesticide. This can combine with our genes and create other proteins that the human body is not yet adapted to deal with. There are increased allergies associated with the introduction of GMO foods, although most of the info about these are kept hidden from us. When GMO corn was introduced into our food supply in the 1990's Monarch butterflies were affected by it. Cornell researchers in 1999, published a study where they fed monarch butterflies, corn pollen full of genetically engineered Bt-corn, and they died. As this book goes to press, most of the Genetic engineering done is to make the plant resist bugs. Some is now done to improve the color or the nutrient yield. But inserting a pesticide genome affects our DNA. It does not enhance the health of the person eating it, however, and may in fact be harmful to us.

Doctors at the Institute of Foreign Trade and Management in Uttarakhand, India. published a review of the research on the effects of animals fed genetically modified foods in 2011. The report was, "Several animal studies indicate serious health risks associated with GM food, including infertility, immune problems, accelerated aging, insulin regulation, and changes to major organs and the GI system."[16]

---

[16] Verma, C., Nanda, K., Singh, R. & Mishra, S. (2011) A review on impacts of genetically modified food on human health. *The Open Nutraceuticals Journal*, 4(1).

Back to your Mexican food plate; What spices do you accent to make it Mexican? Try cumin seeds, cilantro leaves, and chili powder. Or opt for an Adobo mix for that Spanish-Mexican flavor. If you can tolerate red cayenne pepper, substitute it for black. Cayenne has a special ability to cleanse the blood, according to Chinese medicine.[17] Cayenne also fights pain and is used as an ingredient in topical pain relievers some of you may be using.

There are many hot peppers you can experiment with. I'm just too much of a wimp to go near them—jalapeno, habanero, etc.

CELIAC DISEASE, WHAT IT IS:

It is a very serious illness, for those unfamiliar with it. This disease prevents the person with it from consuming any foods containing gluten. Therefore, most people starting on the Celiac diet rely on corn and rice as mainstay grains because they are unfamiliar with the other whole grains and are too exhausted to look into new foods. When someone with Celiac eats a gluten-containing food such as a flour burrito, he becomes very sick because his body has no way to absorb the food. Intestinal cells have become damaged by the gluten. We need finger-like projections, microscopic in size, called *villi* in our intestines to absorb our food to gain energy from it. With Celiac disease, the villi flatten and are unable to wave the way they should to absorb food. The blood and saliva of people with Celiac contain antibodies to the protein components in gluten-containing grains. When our body creates antibodies, it reacts to something it considers foreign and mounts a defense. This could mean the release of histamine commonly observed with Hay fever allergy. In the case of Celiac, the GI tract highlights many of

---

[17] Pitchford, Paul, (2002). Healing with whole foods: Asian traditions and modern nutrition. North Atlantic Books.

the symptoms. This illness currently means a lifetime sentence without wheat, barley, rye, and in some cases, oats. Thus, corn tortillas, rice-based casseroles, tasty rice pasta, and quinoa are the grain foods on which most people with Celiac rely. Once the energy level is regained, people will try amaranth, millet and teff.

The resultant malabsorption from Celiac damage can prevent a child from reaching her true height, cause failure to thrive, abdominal pain, memory and concentration difficulties, as well as balance issues. It can turn into cancer of the small intestine and become life-threatening in some cases, so a diagnosis is important. This illness requires food be prepared using separate cutting boards, and cooking pots as a person can become sick if their non-gluten food even touches something containing gluten. The diet in this book is not aimed at people with Celiac Disease, but you may know of someone who has it.

For those who want the knowledge: Early symptoms of celiac are: memory and concentration problems, followed by weakness, fatigue, weight loss, and diarrhea. Unfortunately, the only treatment (as this goes to press), is to avoid gluten from all sources. No prescription pill can stop your body from reacting to gluten. But there are supplements that make it easier for those with *gluten intolerance*, a related condition, to eat gluten-containing foods. The gluten-free diet used to be a tough diet to follow, but the supermarkets are embracing gluten-free foods these days, including good tasting bread. I haven't found an Italian Scali bread that is GF yet. However, there are crackers, cookies, sauces, condiments, and baking mixes to try. If you are using gluten-free foods, look for those with 3 grams of fiber or more per serving.

I do not have Celiac Disease, but my doctors advised me to follow a restricted gluten diet to increase my energy.

You may know people who, like myself, follow a mostly GF diet because we are gluten-intolerant. This is an allergy to wheat and its main component, gluten.

SEVEN TIPS FOR THE SENSITIVE STOMACH

1. Replace red onions with green ones They are milder and less likely to burn sensitive mucous membranes.
2. Replace white vinegar with more delicate rice wine vinegar or even a sweet balsamic vinegar. White vinegar can be very harsh. Did you know that people wash windows and clean coffee makers with white vinegar?
3. Replace fried chicken and fish with baked. The oil used to fry foods often becomes undigestible.
4. If cultured foods such as yogurt and kefir are new to you, introduce them by the teaspoon. Finicky digestive tracts often react to large amounts of beneficial bacteria found in these that are considered unfamiliar to the GI tract.
5. Avoid artificial colors and preservatives, especially - Sulfite, used for keeping foods white in color. It often causes nausea and asthma attacks.
6. Avoid tight or restricted clothing, including belts. They often push the contents of the stomach upward, contributing to reflux or heartburn.
7. If tomato sauce is too spicy, add a small amount of raw agave nectar, a sweetener, to decrease the acidity.

CHAPTER 6

FROM THE REFRIGERATED CASE

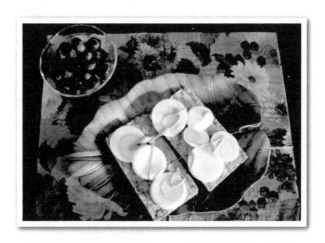

SCRAMBLED SCIENCE OR EGG-CELLENT FOOD?

Nutrient-rich eggs with their unique design, are really neatly packaged protein. And now they are considered good for us! Hurray! For years, eggs were viewed as the villains that cause cholesterol to rise. Now we know that the cholesterol in eggs has no connection to the cholesterol in your body. Even people who have heart disease are allowed to eat 5 eggs per week! I would stick to organic as the feed on conventional chicken farms is full of GMO's that enter the structure of the egg. For decades, eggs sat on the naughty-foods list which is a shame because eggs are the highest biologically available source of protein! Did you know eggs are the standard against which researchers compare other foods? Eggs are full of the protein-building blocks, which we call *amino acids*, needed to keep muscles strong. Each little oval egg, is a complete source of the energy-producing B vitamins we all need, plus two more, *lecithin* and choline. Our brains need the latter for healthy nerve functioning to keep memory sharp. Eggs also provide us with some vitamin E.

Newer research shows a mineral found in eggs, *selenium*, boosts immune function. What a great way to obtain the selenium instead of in supplement form.

Choline found in eggs and other foods is essential for nerve messages to travel from one place in the body to another. When you touch a hot iron, your finger senses the pain and, by way of your nervous system, sends a message to your brain that the iron is hot; you jerk your finger away—hopefully without a burn. This is nerve transmission. For the news to travel, our nerve endings secrete substances called *neurotransmitters*. Choline in the form of lecithin makes up 30% of our brains as well as the neurotransmitter that carries the signal substance, *acetylcholine*. Choline is also a component of the covering wrapped around our spinal cord and brains, the myelin sheath and the *meninges*, respectively.

Those of you with Chronic Fatigue Syndrome may be interested in knowing that in other countries, instead of being referred to as SEID, the illness is referred to as *Myalgic Encephalomyelitis*, a far more accurate name for it, by referring to the inflammation of the myelin covering the brain. The "itis" means inflammation. Therefore, I have included many eggs in this eating program.

You need eggs to keep the vulnerable covering over the nerves intact. Eggs also contain pigments which give their yolks the bright sunny hue, full of *lutein* and *zeaxanthin*, two nutrients that our eyes require to function. These pigments make their way from the egg yolks we eat, to the eye tissues, helping to avoid eye damage from the sun[18] and may help you avoid macular degeneration, a serious condition of the eye that can result in blindness.

Did you know that eggs actually *benefit* our hearts? Due to their choline content, they lower the risk of having high *homocysteine* levels, a risk factor for heart disease. The other animal-derived foods, milk, meat, and cheese, with their saturated fat content, raise cholesterol. According to an extensive review of studies undertaken by Dr. Maria Luz Fernandez of the University of Connecticut,[19] two-thirds of the population at any age can eat two or three eggs every day without affecting their cholesterol!

SLIM-DOWN WITH EGGS

I know there are readers out there who want to find an easy way to lose a few pounds. Well, here is one! Eggs can give you a slimmer waistline. An eight-week study done by researchers from the Pennington Biomedical Research Center in Louisiana compared the waistlines of women given eggs to eat at breakfast to those of women who ate a breakfast of bagels. Both breakfasts had the same calories, but the women who ate two eggs a day, five days a week,

---

[18] Roberts, J. E. & Dennison, J. (2015).The Photobiology of lutein and zeaxanthin in the eye. *Journal of Ophthalmology*. 2015; Dec 20 doi 10.1155/2015/687173
[19] Fernandez, M.L. (2006). Dietary cholesterol provided by eggs and plasma lipoprotein in healthy populations. *Current Opinions in Clinical Nutrition & Metabolic Care*. 9(1), 8-12

achieved smaller waistlines and were more energetic than the bagel eaters! A year later, men joined in the studies, and the results were the same. This time, the information was published in the well-respected *International Journal of Obesity*. Men and women followed a low-calorie diet and started off their day with 2 eggs; they all lost weight.[20] There wasn't just a few pounds lost, but a 65% greater weight loss in the group that received eggs for breakfast!

So how do eggs work their magic? For one, eggs regulate blood sugar more effectively than do carbohydrates such as breads and bagels. Eggs have an anti-inflammatory effect that is effective against heart disease. The B vitamin, Choline, found in eggs, counteracts the effects of the adrenaline and cortisol that our bodies release during stress, thereby keeping the heart rate healthy.

For those who are pregnant or wish to become pregnant, the Folic Acid in eggs prevents congenital conditions like *Spina bifida* from developing in the unborn baby. Purchase organic eggs for the best source of nutrients and to avoid any genetically modified feed given to hens on conventional farms.

FREE RANGE AND ORGANIC

I like to purchase my eggs, either organic or omega-enriched. For the latter, I will gain all the heart-healthy and joint-loving benefits of the omega 3's. For those not familiar with the term, omega-3 oils fed to the hens have powerful anti-inflammatory properties. Anyone with Lyme disease or arthritis will appreciate this effect. Just as the flesh of animals fed omega-3 transfer the benefits to us, so do the eggs from organically-raised hens.

---

[20] Vander Wal, J.S., Gupta, A., Khosla, P., & Dhurandhar, N.V. (2008) Egg breakfast enhances weight loss. *International Journal of Obesity*, 32(10), 1545-1551

Some hens have a good life. They spend the day outdoors casually eating leftover scraps of vegetables and peels, eating a feed rich in omega-3 oils, and basking in the sun. This is the type of environment that an egg from a free-range farm comes from. Similar conditions exist on organic farms. Contrast this to the conventional farm where hens are fed cornmeal rich in omega 6 oils that are pro-inflammatory. In addition, these animals are housed in restricted places and fed the blood and guts of other animals. This gets passed on to the consumer through the eggs. Maybe this adds a new dimension to that old saying, "You are what you eat."

I enjoy my eggs, hard-boiled and ready for use, with shells intact. These can keep for up to a week in the fridge. Boiling half a dozen at one time makes life easier. The secret to getting the shells to glide right off; after cooking plunge them under cold running water, then refrigerate.

Here are four simple ways to combine eggs with veggies:

Add sliced hard boiled eggs to a bed of mixed greens and grated carrot and black olives. Sprinkle with raisins and shredded cheddar cheese.

Zesty mesclun greens drizzled with sweet honey, cucumbers, grape tomatoes combined with chunks of egg makes a tasty salad.

Create a melange of soft velvety greens with Bibb lettuce and crunchy rings of red pepper mixed with the white and yellow orbs of hard boiled eggs. Sprinkle with toasted sunflower seeds for extra vitamin E.

Drizzle a cream-style commercial dressing, one made with olive oil, over slices of egg and surround it with baby spinach and canned mandarin orange segments.

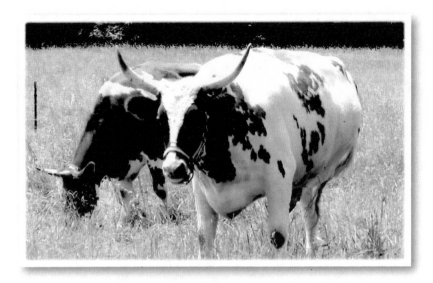

COWS ARE WHAT THEY EAT

Have you ever seen Robert Kenner's documentary, <u>Food, Inc.</u>? It's an eye opener on the practices of conventional dairy farming. Cows are crammed together in stalls, fed genetically-engineered grain full of omega-6 corn and soy—the inflammatory fats. One horror is cows consume other animals' body parts as part of their feed. Farmers use dangerous pesticides in an effort to keep bugs off the cows and inject them with hormones to fatten them for market; cows are given antibiotics to prevent mastitis infections. Not a pretty picture and not good for the health of the consumer eating those products. In addition to these unpleasant situations, animals have been cloned, and the clones are part of our food supply. Of course, there are no labels to tell us the meat we are eating is a clone. I purchase only organic meat, dairy, and poultry to ensure my food is free of antibiotics, hormones, petrochemicals, and to ensure I'm not eating a clone! To confirm the meat I am eating is not coming from an animal fed fattening corn, I look for pasture-raised or free-range beef. This is more important if you buy ground beef for those delicious hamburgers out on the grille. For those of you who are unable to find these options in your markets, you can order free-range beef online. And do not be afraid to talk to the management of your local stores and ask them to provide pasture-raised and free-range meat. Remember, consumer demand is an important element in supply.

Cows do more than provide meat. We learn as children that milk comes from cows. Organic dairy is optimal because the milk from conventional farms contains residue from all the contaminants mentioned above. Also, the taste of organic is better! While it costs more per package, organic cheese is free of all these contaminants, which do not benefit anyone's health, most especially, all of us struggling to keep healthy.

A one-half gallon of non-organic milk in the North East costs approximately $1.75, whereas the organic milk could be $3.99 on sale to $4.50. It costs more, but it's definitely worth it. I also purchase imported cheeses from the European countries that forbid the use of genetically altered enzymes in the making of the cheeses, unlike here in the U.S.A.

Sometimes a cold frosty glass of milk makes a meal complete. Who doesn't enjoy a glass of milk with two chocolate chip cookies now and then? When purchasing milk, I always choose organic. Who wants all those residues of antibiotics and hormones in the milk you drink? The jury is out on what type of milk is best. We are told to consume low- fat varieties, such as skim or 1%. This is fine as long as you don't have an issue with lactose intolerance. For those unfamiliar with this condition, I'll explain.

ARE YOU LACTOSE-INTOLERANT?

We are born with an enzyme, a protein substance, allowing our intestines to digest the milk sugar, lactose. This enzyme just happens to have a name sounding like the sugar that it breaks down, except that, being an enzyme, its suffix is "-ase." Due to a genetic glitch, some members of the human race lose the ability to digest milk products, experiencing gas and bloating when consuming milk products. Whether less enzyme is produced or just becomes less efficient at doing its job, is unknown at present. We know that people with lactose intolerance are better able to tolerate milk and cheese products with a higher fat content because the fat slows down the absorption time.

The other alternative is to purchase milk that contains the lactase enzyme, so the milk is already broken down. (Lactaid is one brand, but it's not available in organic form as of this printing.) This way, you still obtain the necessary nutrients milk and its products provide. We all need calcium, and its partner, phosphorous is found naturally in milk, not in calcium supplements. Milk also provides energy-giving nutrients; the B-vitamin, riboflavin, protein to build muscle tissue and bones, and it has two more important vitamins, A and D. It's far more preferable to receive all these nutrients at the same time in the natural package they come in. Lactaid also can be purchased as a tablet you take when eating or drinking milk products.

A MOUTHFUL OF WORDS: CONJUGATED LINOLEIC ACID (CLA)

The American Heart Association recommends consuming low-fat milk and cheese. However, if you always have low-fat dairy, you may be missing out on a nutrient that can help your heart. Have you ever heard of CLA? Conjugated linoleic acid, is found in the fatty portion of milk from grass-fed cows. Animal studies have found that CLA offers many benefits, according to German research from Munster. CLA may be one of the healthiest omega-6 fats we can consume as it lowers inflammation.[21] The resistance to tumors is one; avoidance of weight-gain is another because CLA increases metabolism by using fat for fuel; a boost to the immune system is a third. CLA decreases the risk of breast, colon, and prostate cancers. It's too early to recommend taking CLA supplements but research is being done to see what effect CLA has on the proliferation of cancerous cells. What we do know is that CLA stops the blood supply created when a tumor grows, in order to feed it. This is exciting news! In the meantime, you can get CLA from *free-range* meat and grass-fed dairy. Often the whole food packaged by nature, offers much more than a single substance purified in a lab and prevents other diseases as well.

If you are looking for another high-protein, calcium-rich beverage, you may enjoy yogurt-based smoothies. Smoothies are basically fruit combined with yogurt made into a creamy beverage. *Stonyfield Farms* offers yummy ones that come in interesting flavors such as, peach, strawberry and strawberry-banana. One of my favorite yogurt beverages is the Mango Lassie I drink at Indian restaurants. This yellow drink is so smooth and refreshing and we get the breast and prostate protection from the mango.

---

[21] Benjamin S., & Spener, F. (2009). Conjugated linoleic acids as functional food: an insight into their health benefits. *Nutrition & Metabolism*, 6(1), 36.

GOT MORE ENERGY TODAY?

Make your own smoothie. Just combine vanilla or unflavored yogurt with a cup of frozen fruit in the blender and add the sweetener of your choice. I use Maple Syrup!

LES POMMES DE TERRE

You can make a meal from a baking potato, broccoli and some meltable cheese. (Recipe will follow). I buy only organic potatoes because this vegetable requires many applications of pesticides when it is grown conventionally. Remember, potatoes grow underneath the ground; so many critters are attracted to them. On the organic farm, the farmers make certain that the soil conditions don't favor potato beetles.

The name for potatoes in France, means 'apples of the earth.' Have you ever noticed how alike are the flesh of the apple and the potato? The pectin of the apple is used to thicken jams and jellies. The starch of the potato is used for thickening soups and sauces.

Potatoes are so versatile; roasted, grilled, boiled, whipped, and baked are just a few ways to enjoy them. Have you ever seen potatoes growing? I had the opportunity of living on an organic farm, and it was the most wonderful experience of my life. I used to go into the fields and dig into the mineral-rich earth to find them. I was literally up to my elbows in the dirt. Because potatoes grow underground, they are a rich source of the minerals found there: potassium, phosphorous, and selenium. Potassium keeps blood pressure healthy. Selenium is an immune system booster. Phosphorous helps build bones. Choline, which you heard about in the egg section, is also found in potatoes and helps our brains retain memory, and decreases inflammation. Since organic soil has not been depleted, more minerals and vitamins are found in the produce grown in it: magnesium, vitamin C, and vitamin B6 (great for PMS and PMD). I buy organic potatoes so I can eat its mineral-rich skin along with the flesh. Because most of the minerals are found in the skin, so when you can, eat the whole package! especially for the fiber. When I choose organic, I have no worries about pesticide residue ending up on my food and my family.

Potatoes are also a good food for building muscle tissue and regulating the amount of acidity in our bodies. Greater acidity is associated with more inflammation, more food allergies, and poorer health. At only 110 calories per potato, they are not fattening at all. Due to its high calcium, phosphorous, and magnesium content, this meal may reduce high blood pressure!

POTATO MEAL:

Cheddar cheese melted over a stalwart baking potato and studded with crunchy broccoli florets.

Ingredients:

> 1 baking potato
>
> 1 stalk of broccoli
>
> 1-2 ounces organic cheese, shredded

1) Wash a raw baking potato under running water, then stab it with the tines of a fork to allow gasses to escape during the baking process.
   1. Bake in the oven for one hour at 425°F.

2) While potato cooks, pour an inch of water into the bottom of a medium pan and steam the broccoli so that it remains crunchy.

3) Once the potato is cooked, add the broccoli florets from the pan and sprinkle with the grated cheese.

4) If you line the baking sheet with aluminum foil, you won't have to wash anything. Return potato, cheese and broccoli to oven, underneath the broiler, just until the cheese bubbles and then browns slightly.

To this meal, let's add a piece of fruit and a cup of tomato juice. Later plan to nibble on a few celery sticks with peanut butter to reach your leafy green allotment as well as gain protein from the peanut butter. For those allergic to peanut butter, try some cashew butter or substitute hummus.

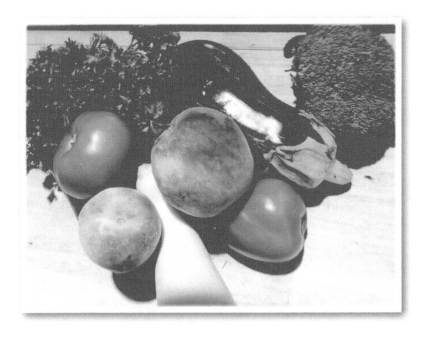

CHAPTER 7

FIGHTER NUTRIENTS
FROM FRUITS AND VEGETABLES

I had a client at one time who told me that she was eating two servings of vegetables every day. When we carefully went over "Gina's" written food diary, we both recognized that the pickle she was having at lunch and the sprig of parsley that decorated her chicken dinner, which she thought were her two servings of vegetables, did not qualify. She knows now that two cups of leafy green spinach and one cup of butternut squash are the two true sources of vegetables. Why do we nutritionists put such enormous emphasis on fruit and veggies?

Think of produce as power cells holding the nutrients our bodies need to function. From them, we obtain electrolytes to keep our hearts beating at a regular pace; fiber, that gets things moving regularly; trace minerals to keep our bones intact; and most importantly, enzymes, which drive the chemical reactions that keep our bodies running smoothly. We also get protective factors in the form of such tongue-tying words as *phyto-chemicals* and anti-oxidants. *"Phyto"* which means plant, refers to the good things that are naturally found inside of plants. Anti-oxidants fight aging and the onslaught of nasty things in our environment called free radicals. We create a defense plan against these "free rads" when we eat many fruits and vegetables.

It probably comes as little surprise to hear most people come to me for counseling, do not eat enough fruit and veggies. A dear friend of mine, died, from continually making poor dietary choices. People who don't eat fruit are unhealthy and have bowel troubles. You see, our bodies were designed to eat plant matter. Not only that, we need to consume a range of between 5 to 13 servings of produce every day. Now I know that sounds daunting, but even the USDA supports this in their guidelines. It was initiated way back in 1991 when the National Cancer Institute (NCI), launched a public awareness campaign called "5 A DAY" to convey to all Americans the importance of eating produce. Following on its heels, the Healthy People 2010, launched by the National Institute of Health, (NIH), published a list of recommended goals for the United States. Included was the goal of increasing daily fruit consumption to TWO servings and vegetables to THREE. A government report disclosed in a publication that tracks statistics of disease interestingly named, *Morbidity and Mortality Weekly*, indicates that less than 32% of Americans achieved the goal of having 3 vegetables every day.[22] Not one state in the entire country met the goals of the Healthy People 2010. Things became worse: The same publication printed a drearier picture of what Americans eat with a 2017 report that the number of people meeting the goal decreased to 10%.[23] No

---

[22] Grimm, K.A., Blanck, H.M., Scanlon, K.S., Moore, L.V., Grummer-Strawn, L.M., & Foltz, J.L. (2010).State-specific trends in fruit and vegetable consumption among adults-United States, 2000-2009. *Morbidity and Mortality Weekly Report*, 59(35), 1125-1130

[23] CDC Press Releases 2016, January 1). Retrieved from http://www.cdc.gov/media/releases/2017/p1116-fruit-vegetable-consumption-html

wonder we need allergy pills and laxatives. We aren't eating the bulk we need or the nutrients our bodies require to stay healthy! Of course, a 2020 goal ensued, and now we look to the 2030 guidelines.

Reflecting on what I just talked about, one of the Healthy People 2030 goals are . . . wait for it . . . "Increase consumption of dark green vegetables, red and orange vegetables, and beans and peas by people age 2 years and older." The Office of Disease prevention got very specific here and this is my aim throughout this book; to help you reach this goal as well.

PRODUCE PACKS A POWERFUL PUNCH!

Eating adequate fruits and vegetables is a no-brainer for some of us. Those are the people who realize fruits and vegetables can do amazing things for us. Who doesn't wish to have healthy, radiant skin? Eating adequate produce hydrates us. Also, the fluids we drink and the fiber in produce assures us a regular pattern of pooping. It assures our bodies' improved toxin removal resulting in more energy. More good news: some people when eating a very high produce intake, were actually able to throw away their high blood pressure pills! Amazing, don't you think?

I am referring to the D.A.S.H Diet which stands for Dietary Approaches to Stop Hypertension eating plan. It was found to be as successful at lowering blood pressures as well as the pills from the pharmacy. However, it can be a challenge, as it requires eating 9 to 11 servings of fruit and vegetables every day. Once you start eating this way, you will feel so good you won't want to eat any other way. You will have variety, color, all the minerals and vitamins you need plus all the antioxidants as well.

We have accumulated massive amounts of oxidative stress, (analogous to rust build up) inside our cells and joint tissues, causing pain and fatigue. We need phytonutrients to fuel our ailing bodies, and fruits and vegetables are the way to obtain the majority of them. These are not found in milk and meat products. An easy way to remember what they do for us is to think of "Phyto" sounding like 'fight" so we can increase our immune systems' productivity. Many fatiguing illnesses involve abnormalities of the immune systems where the B and T cells, specialized cells that fight the invaders, do not work or are produced adequately.

If you suffer from an autoimmune condition, you too require a variety of nutrients and specific fats, from Extra Virgin Olive oil, fish and nuts, to keep inflammation from taking over.

Our campaign is to increase the number of our T cells used to fight minor sinus infections, or that urinary tract infection and enlarge the capacity of our natural killer cells (NK) to destroy tumor cells that may be lurking. You might be tempted to do this with supplements, but it won't have the same effect and can be harmful by throwing off the natural balance of things. Whole, unadulterated foods, on the other hand, will maintain balance. Take an orange, for example, a complete package of nutrients with all the cofactors and enzymes needed to digest it. You receive *quercetin* from that white part that clings to the flesh as well as vitamin C and the fiber that all work together. When you extract these nutrients and place them inside a pill or capsule, something gets lost.

We need Phytonutrients, found in water-soluble foods and the poly sterols found in the avocado. When I stock my fridge with healthy juice, fruits and vegetables, I am careful to check the temperature, to keep it low enough to keep harmful bacteria from multiplying. That would be 41 degrees for the fridge and 0 degrees for the freezer. It is well worth the money to purchase an inexpensive thermometer made specifically for this purpose.

Let me get up on my soap box for a moment with my megaphone. "9-to-11" servings of fruits and vegetables is the goal. Some of you may have felt sicker when increasing your produce intake - but ask yourself this question? Was it organic? Because many of us react to even the smallest trace of pesticides found in conventional produce; it is worth trying once again. You may not react with organic choices. Wait until you taste the difference! Organic produce is sweeter and often has a finer texture than conventionally grown. The bitter taste that some pesticides leave behind, is absent in the organic produce. The only downside with organic is the produce may be smaller in size. Remember, we want to flood our tissues with antioxidants from food.

If you can tolerate it, eat as many organic fruits, raw, with their enzymes still intact as you possibly can. Chosen because they require little preparation, you'll find a list of fruits in this chapter. If you use any of the NSAIDS, which many rely on for pain control, you could be at risk of getting ulcers or small holes in your stomach and small intestine. What if you could reduce that risk with a simple eating habit? Good News!

Data from the Health professional Follow-up Study proved that fruits and vegetables delay emptying of the stomach contents into the intestines, thereby preventing the development of these erosions in the first part of the small intestine; duodenal ulcers.[24]

THE DIRTY DOZEN

Do you know what is in your food? Do you purchase mostly organic fruits and vegetables? We are the group that most needs to

---

[24] Papas, M.A., Giovanucci, E., & Platz, E.A. (2004). Fiber from fruit and colorectal neoplasia. *Cancer Epidemiology and Prevention Biomarkers*, 13(8), 1267-1270.http://cebp.aactjournalis.org/content/13/8/1267

know what may be lurking in our food supply. One of the things we most want to avoid is . . . pesticides! Exposure to a certain class of pesticides, known as *"organochlorines"* can actually decrease our natural killer cells' activity.[25] Are you aware that metabolites of pesticides are found in the urine when we eat conventional produce? The non-profit Environmental Working Group (EWG), using data compiled by the USDA and the FDA, creates an annual list of produce found to have the highest proportion of pesticides when tested. They call these *'The Dirty Dozen.'* These types of produce are found to contain *significant* amounts of pesticides throughout the entire flesh, not merely in the rind or skin. Since the deadly chemicals infiltrate the fruit or vegetable's flesh throughout its entire growth period, rinsing has little benefit. Not only do pesticides get into food from the soil, but they also persist in our bodies, especially in fatty tissues such as the breasts, prostate, and brain! If your wallet will not stretch far enough to purchase all organic produce, be sure to purchase these in organic form.

Produce to Purchase in Organic Form	
apples	peaches
cherries	cantaloupe
grapes	spinach
lettuce	strawberries
nectarines	sweet bell peppers
celery	cucumbers

---

[25] Racciatti, D., Vecchiet, J., Ceccomancini, A., Ricci, F., & Pizzigallo, E. (2001). Chronic fatigue syndrome following a toxic exposure. *Science of the total environment*, 270(1-3), 27-31.

To this list, I add zucchini, corn, white potatoes, and broccoli. All of these have been getting genetically altered, and the frozen form of butternut squash is loaded with pesticide residue. Potatoes are prone to both bugs and fungus, making them difficult to grow, so I purchase only organic white potatoes. If you have any immune dysfunction or deficiency, you will want to steer clear of pesticides! With an ever-increasing amount of people under the age of 4o, being diagnosed with colon and rectal cancers, we need to be super vigilant about what we consume. It may turn out that genetic engineering combined with pesticides are to blame for these illnesses.

THE FRUIT BASKET

The old saying, "An apple a day keeps the Doctor away," even to this day, remains a valid statement; as long as you choose organic apples because apples, abound in the soluble fiber, *pectin*. This fiber lowers cholesterol and satisfies hunger. You'll find abundant minerals: potassium which lowers blood pressure and boron, which keeps calcium inside our bones. The three grams of fiber found in an apple with its skin also help to speed the transit time of food in the lower digestive tract preventing constipation. Don't throw away the peel of that organic apple—it contains valuable nutrients such as quercetin just like the orange.

Even more good news about apples! In a study carried out at Florida State University, Women given apples to eat every day for a year had improvements in their good and bad cholesterol, and a reduction in a protein-marker of inflammation referred to as *C-reactive protein* (CRP). This is one of those things your doctor tests you for because CRP becomes elevated in several illnesses including rheumatoid and some heart conditions and cancers.

Apples contain flavonoids, called *phenolics*, which Researchers at Cornell have found will decrease human colon cancer cells' activity.[26] It will also lower cholesterol in rats. Well, since we are not rats, let's hope some of this positive effect extends to the human species. If you are one of those people who cannot digest raw apple, heat slices of it in a mixture of coconut oil and cinnamon. You may find it easier to digest in its cooked form.

Bananas are full of vitamin B6, important for our nervous system. By now everyone is aware of the high potassium found in bananas, but they're full of other goodies such as Vitamin B6, which calms the nervous system, and another mineral, magnesium. My clients have found it most helpful for premenstrual disorders to eat bananas. This fruit has a unique property in being able to regulate the water content in our intestines, whether stopped up or running too much. Part of the B.R.A.T. diet, one commonly used to control diarrhea, bananas actually regulate intestinal motility, helping to clear up diarrhea and its opposite, constipation.

BERRIES - THE SUPER FOOD!

Of all kinds, Berries are superfoods, jam-packed with antioxidants that offer an array of benefits. Chief among them are *ellagic acid* which stops cancer cells from dividing, and *anthocyanins* which lower the blood pressure and exert anti-inflammatory effects. Berries prevent cognitive impairment and an eye disease, and macular degeneration. Berries are low in calories, less than 80 calories per cup. They prevent cell damage, are high in fiber, and the darker hues protect our eyes from an *acute macular degeneration* (AMD). This is a serious eye disease that can impair vision and lead

---

[26] Rana, S., & Bhushan, S. (2016). Apple phenolics as nutraceuticals: assessment, analysis and application. *Journal of food science and technology*, 53(4), 1727-1738.

to blindness when the macula part of the eye actually fails to receive the nutrients and oxygen it needs.

In particular, Strawberries have been found to decrease inflammation[27] according to a 2011 study found in the British Journal of Nutrition and appear helpful in regulating sugar in those with diabetes.[28]

Aim for a half cup of blueberries, blackberries, or strawberries every day. You may wish to try Goji and Acai berries, both with very high antioxidant protective factors, which are gaining popularity. During the time of flu and Covid, another berry, elderberry, strengthens the immune system. You can drink it as a tea or take it in capsules and syrups.

Look for unsweetened jams made from these beneficial berries in your supermarket—delicious when spread on rice or rye crackers. Good on whole wheat crackers for those of you haven't any issues with wheat flour. Anyone battling gum disease? Berries have the benefit of Co-Enzyme Q10, which reduces the incidence of gum disease. Many of us are using medications that cause dry mouth as a side effect. Did you know that dry mouth puts us at higher risk of gum disease? Bacteria responsible for periodontal disease or gingivitis find the desert-like condition of a dry mouth an attractive environment and want to settle there. You'll aways find me carrying a water bottle throughout the year, to keep these problems at bay.

---

[27] Gao, Q., Qin, L. Q., Arafa, A., Eshak, E.S.,& Dong, J.Y. (2020) Effects of strawberry intervention on cardiovascular risk factors: A meta-analysis of randomised controlled trials. *British Journal of Nutrition*; 124(3):241-2246. http://doi:10.1017/S000711452000121X

[28] Calvano, A., Izuora, K., Oh, E.C.,Ebersole, J.L., Lyons, T.J., & Basu, A. (2019)Dietary berries, insulin resistance, and type 2 diabetes: an overview of human feeding trials. *Food & function*, 10(10), 6227-6243 doi.10.1039/c9fo01426h

CITRUS FRUIT

Juicy Citrus fruit: clementines, tangerines, mandarin oranges, grapefruit, and pomelos quench thirst and are full of color with their orange rind and yellow flesh. Clementines, oranges, and grapefruit with their white bitter-tasting pith, overflow in quercetin—a natural anti-histamine. This amazing nutrient prevents certain cells in our bodies (mast cells) from releasing all of the gunk that stops up the sinus or makes eyes weak and weepy. The great part about Citrus fruit is they require no more preparation than removing the rind; they boast of vitamin C which boosts the immune system and aids in cell repair. In this group, we must include lemons and limes that always look attractive piled in a glass bowl. Maybe you're one of those who enjoy eating these sour fruits, which make my mouth pucker. Many of us squeeze the juice from them to add to apples and pears to keep them from browning, while making apple pies and pear tarts. Lemons and limes are good for seasoning fish, and limes are important in making salsa and even can be used in place of salad dressing.

Embraced by the Greek culture, lemons are frequently added to food. Have you ever had Greek chicken lemon soup (*avgolemono*)? It's a creamy version of chicken soup instead of clear broth and soothing and delicious. Citrus fruit has some interesting properties relevant to our overly challenged GI tracts. The weak acid in them forms a citrate in the stomach, helping to neutralize stomach acid. I remember as a child, watching my grandmother use lemon-flavored Brioschi to settle her stomach. You can find this effervescent product at Walmart.com. Italian markets sell something similar, called, *Galeffi Effervescente*, which is crystals you place in water then you drink it as it fizzes.

During infections and the stress of battling chronic illness, including the Covid19 that some of you are fatigued and hurting from, our adrenal glands consume greater quantities of vitamin C, which we can easily obtain from vitamin-C rich fruits and vegetables. One of the deficiency symptoms of this vitamin is cracking in the corners of the mouth or lips. If you have this, you may need to avoid citrus as it tends to sting the area. Using a straw may be helpful. Citrus fruit is naturally low in fat and high in fiber, which is also a source of folic acid and important for DNA repair as well as for a host of other reasons.

Kiwi fruit, juicy green orbs hidden inside their fuzzy tan coats, are sweet and crammed with vitamin C, fiber, potassium and eye-loving pigments; *lutein* and *zeaxanthin*. These polyphenols are essential to eye health. Kiwis are easy to eat; just cut them in half, and eat with a spoon. Shown to *prevent* a decline in lung function, foods high in vitamin C are important when you have Covid19 or any other lung condition such as asthma or bronchitis. Researchers theorize it may prevent asthma from turning into a more serious and chronic illness called COPD or Chronic Obstructive Pulmonary Disease. This vitamin exerts a protective effect on airway cells and prevents scarring of the respiratory passages.

FROM THE VINEYARDS

Grapes are loaded with the nutrient, *Resveratrol*, also found in red wine. You may wonder as I did, why only red? During wine-making parties, after everyone has stomped all over the grapes (only kidding) to crush the skins of the grapes, if red wine is made, the skins are left in. For white wine, the skins are skimmed out of the mixture. But the benefits in the skin, confirmed by European studies, confirm a lower incidence of heart disease. This is great news for <u>men</u> who like to drink wine. For women, we are best avoiding even one drink of wine per day as it ups our cancer risk.

Maybe women are just better off nibbling red grapes for now. Resveratrol delays the aging of skin cells so supplements are available.

TOTING ENERGY FRUITS!

Dried fruits have greater amounts of nutrients than their fresh counterparts, owing to the water having been removed during the dehydration process, giving us more energy in the form of calories. Dates and figs are two powerhouses of nutrients, such as iron and potassium. Iron is the pigment that carries oxygen to all our cells. Easy-to-eat, mahogany-colored dates and amber figs are chewy and require no preparation unless you wish to soak them to use in recipes. Because dried fruits are a concentrated source of energy, you need to watch how many you eat. You don't eat them like M&M's. However, they are a simple source of minerals. For a treat, I buy dates rolled in banana flakes from my Whole Foods store or dip them into wheat germ or ground flaxseed. Did you know that three medium dates supply you 10 grams of fiber? Enjoy!

Dried cranberries are a versatile food, rich in vitamin C and quite bitter without being sweetened. You can eat the commercially sold, Craisins like raisins that they resemble. I enjoy them as snacks, baked into cookies, added to my rice or Quinoa, or sprinkled on my breakfast cereals. I add them to the cereals that need a boost in flavor or texture. Amaranth flakes come to mind.

Dried plums or prunes, (they can't seem to make up their mind about what they want to be called) are overflowing in potassium and fiber. Time to bust a myth: Although hospitals cook them in water, also called 'stewed,' I prefer to eat them dried and shriveled, sort of like a giant raisin! They get their laxative rep because of their high concentration of sorbitol, a fruit sugar, that draws water into the intestine, which prevents internal logjams. Easily purchased in either a canister or bag, you may enjoy eating 4 or 5 at a sitting. Because I am decreasing my intake of preservatives, I purchase the sorbate-free ones at my Trader Joe's store.

FROM THE TROPICS TO YOUR TABLE

Succulent tropical fruits, with their rich stores of Beta Carotene, such as mangoes, pineapples, and papayas, are delicious, colorful fruit with special properties. Let's start with mango, its brightly colored yellow flesh is very protective of breast and prostate tissues. For a change of pace, I freeze the golden flesh of mango chunks with the indigo orbs of blueberries, eating them as they defrost. Sprinkling coconut flakes on blueberries and mandarin orange segments is one tasty dessert.

Purchase coconut flakes from the store's natural food section, as they are free of the preservative, *metabisulfite*. Most supermarket coconut flakes are treated with sulfites, to keep them white. This preservative has a tendency to cause respiratory symptoms in some people. It can bring on asthma attacks, as it's a respiratory irritant, so if you picked up this book because you had Covid19, be very careful to avoid any form of sulfite! Instead of bringing on full-blown asthma attacks, sulfites on my grapes made me feel extremely worn out. Many dried fruits in an effort to keep them from turning brown, including bananas, papayas, pineapples, apples and pears, are sprayed with this preservative. In fact, you will find it in *most* packages of dried fruit, trail mix, and on some fresh fruit. Grapes are commonly sprayed with sulfites when they are not grown organically.

As I daydream about my someday visit to a Caribbean island, I picture coconut and palm trees on the beach. Food from the

Caribbean islands features small amounts of coconut along with cherries. Did you know that coconut can be beneficial? For years, coconut oil was maligned because it was believed that it was harmful to the heart. Newer research confirms it is healthy. It's often added to shampoos and conditioner for great-looking hair. Eaten, coconut has both anti-bacterial and anti-viral properties from the lauric acid found inside the coconut.

Orange-fleshed Papaya, rich in beta-carotene, is a source of Vitamin A and stimulates sluggish intestines with its fiber, but it also benefits our digestive tracts in another way. Papaya contains a natural digestive enzyme, *papain,* which breaks down foods that tend to be harder to digest, like meat. Some cultures prize eating the black seeds in the center. You may have seen peach-colored tablets of papaya enzyme sold in health food stores, which aid in the digestion of protein foods such as meat which take longer to digest. I am not too patient about cleaning and slicing a papaya, so I prefer to purchase papaya slices in jars for the convenience.

Papaya's mate, pineapple, also offers natural digestive assistance with its bromelain. Pineapple is also another source of vitamin C. Both contain digestive enzymes and are offered in many European restaurants as dessert. Try a Brazilian Buffet sometime, and you will enjoy skewers of grilled pineapple, served alongside the meats. It's the bromelain in pineapple that is especially helpful in digesting meat. Serve your family some pre-sliced pineapple rings or chunks the way they do in Chinese restaurants when cooking beef or pork dishes. Below is the chart of fruits I recommend when you begin my program. These have been chosen for their convenience. It is not going to harm you in any way if you choose fruit that does not come from this list.

To this list we add limes/lemons useful for seasoning or eating.

Convenient Fruits for Phase 1

apples	pears
banana	blackberries
frozen or fresh blueberries	cherries
clementines	elderberries
gooseberries	grapes, red or green
dried figs	dates
dried cranberries	kiwis
peaches	plums
dried plums	pre-cut melons
pre-cut pineapple	nectarines
oranges	pomegranate juice
raspberries	strawberries

Convenient-to-Use Vegetables

artichoke hearts	arugula	bamboo sprouts	Bibb lettuce
Boston lettuce	broccoflower	broccoli sprouts	broccoli
cauliflower (frozen, fresh)	carrots (baby/ frozen)	canned pumpkin	celery sticks (buy organic)
cherry tomatoes	Chinese cabbage	cole slaw mix without dressing	cooked beets from a jar
corn on the cob	Edamame (frozen, fresh)	Fennel (Anise)	frozen organic corn
frozen diced peppers	frozen green beans	frozen corn kernels organic	frozen edamame
frozen peas	frozen or fresh snow peas	frozen or fresh spinach (buy organic)	grape tomatoes
sliced mushrooms	spinach, fresh or frozen organic	sweet potatoes	tomato sauce
water chestnuts	watercress	white or yellow potatoes (buy organic only)	yams

Others:

- minced garlic that comes in a jar
- toasted minced garlic
- frozen onions, diced or whole
- dried onion flakes

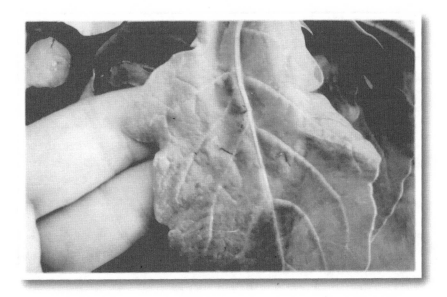

GREENS-A POWER HOUSE OF NUTRIENTS

We need green, leafy vegetables in our diets more than anyone else does, even if some of you begin to grow whiskers and develop long floppy ears. Just the way plants require chlorophyll in order to grow; we humans require chlorophyll for good health. This compound is what gives green foods and even the leaves on trees their green color. In humans, it floods every cell of our bodies with oxygen. Eaten raw or cooked, we all need chlorophyll-rich greens and there are so many good reasons to eat them. They are loaded with the nutrients that give us clear skin, while having little or no fat. They also supply us with some fiber as well as water. They are not however, just for dieters.

Men consuming vegetables full of Beta-carotene found in the leafy greens as well as vegetables such as carrots and squash may be protected from developing an enlarged prostate gland.[29] Some of my clients have reported that their stomachs won't tolerate leafy green lettuce. Here's my theory: It could be that rather than having an intolerance to the greens, these people are reacting to the rocket fuel or perchlorate that contaminates many water supplies. It seeps into the ground water and subsequently, the water we drink, from military bases where it's used for rocket-firing and in flares.[30] This has also been found in many municipal water supplies so a water filter in the kitchen is a healthy choice to use for rinsing. The perchlorate at high levels, can prevent the uptake of iodine by the thyroid gland.

Greens contain the super-mineral, selenium, used by the immune system with cancer-prevention qualities. The green leafies contain tumor-preventing carotenoids such as *lutein* and *zeaxanthin*; you may remember they are pigments that protect our eyes from developing cataracts and macular degeneration. And the great news is that you NEED that fatty dressing in order to absorb all those goodies from the greens! A salad with an olive oil-based dressing will provide us with vitamins, E, A and K. I prefer to use a high-grade olive oil such as EVOO, (extra virgin olive oil). It lacks the contaminants found in the inferior grades such as the misleadingly named, "pure olive oil" or those called "light" while providing a ton of benefits. Now you'd be surprised how little a serving size appears to be. It's a great deal less than what most

---

[29] Kolonel, L.N., Hankin, J.H., Whittemore, A.S., Wu, A.H., Gallagher, R.P., Wilkens, L.R.,...& Paffenbarger, R.S. (2000). Vegetables, fruits, legumes and prostate cancer: a multiethnic case-control study. *Cancer Epidemiology and Prevention Biomarkers*, 9(8), 795-804.

[30] Murray, C.W., Egan, S.K., Kim, H., Beru, N., & Bolger, P.M. (2008). U.S. food and drug administration's total diet study: Dietary intake of perchlorate and iodine. *Journal of Exposure science and Environmental Epidemiology 18, 571-580*

people use at the salad bar. Would you believe one tablespoon is a serving? I know it seems like such a tiny amount to some of you. Start gradually reducing the amount from the half-cup of dressing that people normally use. You will get used to it.

As I mentioned earlier, I steer clear of eating iceberg lettuce because it lacks many of the nutrients that the darker green varieties' nutrients. Some of my clients find it easier to digest greens when they are cooked instead of raw. So load up your soup bowls with cooked greens. More than any other people, we need greens as they are filled with the minerals required for greater health. Those of us with Fibromyalgia or post-polio syndrome realize the value of a relaxed muscle. Romaine and the other green leafies contain minerals such as calcium, which helps muscles to contract and relax.

For stir-fries, I use peanut and sesame oils, which offer a distinctive Asian taste and take longer to start smoking up the kitchen. We call this having a higher smoke point. You may wish to try using sweet Coconut oil, which is starting to return like the phoenix from the ashes. It's now recognized for its anti-bacterial qualities and its ability to boost our immune systems. I sauté my kale or collard green strips in coconut oil for a change of pace.

Leafy greens, including kale, arugula, and watercress, have additional nutrients that lettuce lacks. They are awash in tumor-preventing compounds called *isothiocyanate*s. (That's quite a mouthful, isn't it?). However, it can be easily added to a soup or broth during the last five minutes of cooking. Later you may wish to add collard greens and Swiss chard to your diet. The reasons I recommend having them later is due to their have thick, indigestible ribs in the center of the leaves and stems that require cutting. They are delicious sautéed in coconut or olive oil with a smidgen of garlic. Arugula, a peppery leafy green, is in the *isothionate* family. When I choose this green, I snip the leaves with kitchen scissors rather than chopping it on a cutting board that hurts my neck. The sharp pungent leaves complement hearty bean soups, and remember, beans are abundant in the vitamin, folate, plus the minerals that keep calcium inside our bones.

Are you aware that the bed rest combined with the steroids many of us take, puts us at risk of *osteoporosis?* That's the brittle bone disease caused by calcium being sucked right out of the bones? It does unkind things to the body, causing hips to fracture and the spine to bend out of shape, and it's responsible for 140,000 nursing home admissions in the U.S every year.[31]

Another mineral, often forgotten is Boron. I make sure that I eat enough boron-rich produce, which may offset the use of steroids. Boron is found in many different foods. Among them are crunchy apples, pears, nuts, and juicy grapes, red, green, and purple. I have designed the eating plan, crammed with foods rich in both boron and magnesium, from - vegetables, nuts, and fruit.

Also recognized as essential for bone health is vitamin D3. vitamin D, referred to as *cholecalciferol*, is known as the sunshine vitamin. For those living south of the equator, getting vitamin D through the sun's rays is not difficult, but for those living in North America, we only receive six months of direct sun exposure every year. Those with darker skin containing more melanin are even at higher risk because darker skin creates less vitamin D. Vitamin D helps our bones to absorb calcium. Are you aware that vitamin D3 goes beyond simple bone health? It boosts the immune system so that tumors won't develop. How much vitamin D should we supplement with?

---

[31] Melton III, L.J., (2003). Adverse outcomes of osteoporotic fractures in the general population. *Journal of Bone and Mineral Research*, 18(6), 1139-1141

The number varies by age.[32] According to the NIH, infants require 400 international units or IU per day; 600 IU for anyone ages 1 to 70; and after that, the recommendation changes to 800 IU per day. Pregnant women require 600 IU. The Endocrine Society, however, recommends a much higher amount for all age groups: 1500 - 2000 IU per day for adults and 1000 IU for children and adolescents. My preference is for 1000 IU per day.

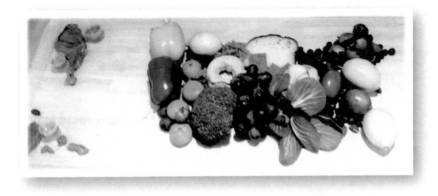

---

[32] Office of Dietary Supplements -Vitamin D. (n.d.) Retrieved from https://ods.od/nih.gov/factsheets/Vitamin D--Health Professional/

CHAPTER 8

THE GEOGRAPHY OF FOOD

THE THREE CONTINENTS OF THE FOOD WORLD

All the foods that we eat can be divided into three main groups, which you can view as the three food continents of the food world. These are fats, proteins, and carbohydrates—often referred to as simply, (carbs). Many of us are familiar with the restriction of diets, such as the South Beach and Keto diets. Beware of any diet that restricts or eliminates any of these food groups because in order to have a well-functioning body, we require all three. However, we don't need the same amount of each. These compounds are created from chains of carbon molecules with hydrogen and oxygen atoms attached.

FAT

Let's start with fat, pictured as the little pools of oil, which often has a bad rap. Fat in the human body can be gross to look at. Have you ever seen it? Decades ago, Oprah took it onstage in a wagon during one of her shows. Big blubbery mounds of yellow stuff. Fat in the diet has been shunned by dieters for years, because it provides 9 calories per gram, containing twice the amount of calories that protein and carbohydrates offer. They only contain 4 grams of Calories per gram. Fat however, is not some waste product hanging around the body. It's a very active substance. The fat that deposits around our middles is actually dangerous because it secretes hormones that can throw off our hormone balance; hormones such as testosterone, estrogen and progesterone. On the opposite extreme, cutting too far back on fat puts us at risk of serious disease. Without enough fat, we would not be able to produce the vital hormones our body makes, nor the fat that pads our internal organs. Fat also makes up our brain matter and plays a role in reproduction. A woman who is too slender, often finds it hard to become pregnant. And being obese, can also cause fertility issues. It is the *type* of fat we consume that makes all the difference. We need the fats that do not promote inflammation in our diets to keep our skin and joints healthy. In fact the lack of certain fats is increasingly linked to forms of arthritis, heart disease, and even cancer!

Americans, in general, consume too many omega-6 fats, from corn and soybean oils, rather than the omega-3 our bodies need to manufacture hormones. That bottle of oil you may have in your house, called "vegetable oil" contributes to your husband's heart disease and your joint pain. It's made from a combination of canola, soybean and corn, none of which are healthy for us. You may find it hard to believe this, but the average American consumes 16 X more inflammation-causing omega-6 fats, than the healthy anti-inflammatory omega-3's. Like a hitch-hiker, fat accompanies other foods. It may be baked into the cookies you buy at the bakery, made with margarine; or it may be a naturally-occurring part of the food—like that crispy chicken skin. Many restaurants, use this oil and you will find many baked goods, cookies, crackers, most of the salad dressings, frozen dinners, and junk food available in supermarkets, contain these oils. Could this be why so many people have joint inflammation, heart disease, cancer, or are overweight? My eating plan for you contains fish, and healthy cold-pressed olive oil from healthy omega 3 fats, including those from grass-fed and free-range dairy and meat. When your diet consists of more omega-3 fats, not only will inflammation no longer be welcome in your body, but your hormones will become more balanced; and your energy level will skyrocket!

THE MAINLAND

We can view carbohydrates as the mainland, with 60 to 75% of our food supply coming from there. *"Carbo-land"* is very colorful with the browns and whites of whole grains, the green and yellows, as well as the red and oranges of the fruits and vegetables that make up this continent. Notice the bell peppers, strawberries, and Bok choy, in the photo. These are not the "bad" guys either that some dietary plans make them out to be. We just need to be selective about what type of carbohydrates we consume.

Found in many of the foods we need to eat, including whole-grain cereals and breads, vegetables, and fruits, "carbs" provide us with the vitamins and minerals required for chemical reactions to take place inside our bodies. The fiber we need to lower our cholesterol, sweep out toxins, and feed the probiotic bacteria living in our intestines—is found in the carbohydrate foods from the Mainland.

Carbohydrates do not require a complicated digestion process. As you learned in chapter 4, simple carbs, such as white crackers, are broken down by salivary amylase right in the mouth. They don't need the strong secretions of the stomach to be digested. This is why, when we are sick with a stomach but, the first solid food we introduce into our system, is plain crackers. Simple carbohydrate foods break down into sugar for quick energy and our brains and muscles require this sugar or glucose as their fuel.

THE ISLES OF PROTEIN

You can envision Protein as islands, such as the Hawaiian Islands, (there I go again with my Hawaiian daydreams). Found in such foods as meat, poultry, and eggs, this group has had the green light for too many years, turning into a most overly consumed food group in the U.S. mostly due to portion sizes, which are just too large for our liver and kidneys to break down. Proteins differ from carbs and fats because the inhabitants that make up this continent are nitrogen, phosphorous, and sulfur groups. These elements are needed to build cells and tissues. In order to break proteins down into their amino acids, the complex digestive process requiring enzymes and hydrochloric acid (HCl), is needed along with a great deal of chewing and mechanical pulverization.

Without enough protein being absorbed, hair, skin, and nails, suffer, along with energy and fluid balance. You have probably seen pictures of starving children In undeveloped countries where severe protein deficiencies are common, the belly starts to protrude as it accumulates fluid.

Phosphorous, another resident of "protein land" is important in creating and maintaining tissues, such as: muscle, bone, and teeth, but not in large amounts. In fact, very little protein is really needed by the average person. The mineral, sulfur, found in protein foods, is extremely important for us. It is used in the liver's detoxification pathways to transform elements not considered beneficial into less toxic compounds. In people with chronic illness with fatigue as a major component, the body may not be utilizing sulfur correctly. Perhaps the pathway has become defective. This is why some people receive enormous benefit for pain by taking the sulfur compound, *Methyl Sufonlyl Methane* (MSM). It supplies the sulfur needed to break things down so that they don't accumulate in tissues, causing pain and preventing oxygen from getting into our tissue. A tissue starved of oxygen will cramp and cause pain.

As far back as 2005, the USDA began recommending that Americans cut down the serving size of meat to 5 1/2 ounces per day. According to the World Cancer Research Fund, "there is strong evidence that consumption of red meat, as well as processed meat, increases the risk of colorectal, nasopharyngeal, stomach and pancreatic cancers."[33] That year was also when cloned animals were added to our food supply. So, the protein needs of people with chronic illness, who are frequently fighting infections; using steroid medications; taking anti-depressant medicines; and losing muscle tissue due to inactivity and the disease itself, are GREATER, in order to maintain lean muscle tissue. Instead of ordering the 16-ounce steak, we need to find plant sources of the extra protein that don't *heme* iron that can turn into deadly nitrosamines.

The changes to the USDA food pattern recommendations were made due to the relationship between eating a diet containing saturated fats, heart disease, and many cancers, including breast and colorectal, from a diet high in these. By eating a plant protein source such as legumes, I know my protein is providing me with antioxidants and fiber, and I receive protective benefits that I would not receive from animal products. Have a side dish of baked

---

[33] World Research Cancer Fund UK. (n.d.) *International* http://www.wcrf.org/

beans purchased from the health food section that doesn't contain corn syrup, to furnish 10 more grams of fiber.

Back to the analogy of the islands! We need more of the island-type residents to strengthen us against infections and create antibodies and white blood cells that fight infection, but we can get this from peanut butter instead of hamburger. Too much protein also affects our kidney function. These two organs located in our backs, filter substances in the blood, and turn it into the waste product that we know of as "urine." One, of these, nitrogen, can tax the kidneys already overloaded from all the medications we are taking. Acetaminophen usage can cause a strain on the kidneys. Years of taking ibuprofen, another popular over the counter pain reliever, can do a job on the stomach lining, setting us up for ulcers. Sensitivities to medications are common in people with chronic illness, especially in those with fibromyalgia and CFIDS. Don't be shy about asking for a lower dose of medications to accommodate your chemistry.

Part of my job as a nutritionist is to teach behavioral strategy to my clients. We work on making small changes from one week to the next. Did you know that it takes the average person 38 days to incorporate a change into his behavior, so that he no longer needs to think about it? That is a month plus eight more days, so be easy on yourself if it doesn't happen overnight. Tiny steps add up to great changes. The trick to being successful is not making too many changes at one time. If eating organically is new to you and difficult on your wallet, make only ONE change per month. The following chart gives an example of a 6-month goal setting plan based on the changes you made in the book's first seven chapters.

GOAL SETTING CHART

- **Month 1:** Try a whole grain bread you have never tried before, such as Kamut, Spelt, or Whole Rye crackers.

- **Month 2:** Buy instant organic oatmeal, which has less sugar, and no preservatives.

- **Month 3:** Make the switch to organic dairy products.

- **Month 4:** Purchase more fruits that are organic. Not only do they provide better nutrients, but they also taste much better!

- **Month 5:** Add more free-range and organic eggs to your breakfast.

- **Month 6:** Eat more legumes or try them if you are unfamiliar with them.

YOGURT UP - TO MEET THE REQUIREMENTS

Everyone has heard of the phrase, "three square meals a day." However, there is no reason why you can't eat two healthy snacks between smaller meals. Those of you with hypoglycemia probably eat more than three meals. You can balance the use of convenience foods with healthy snacks eaten throughout the day. I purchase pre-cut celery and carrot sticks then immerse them in a pitcher filled with water, which I keep in my fridge. You need to buy the celery organic because it is on the dirty dozen list due to pesticide residue. I buy dried herbs or a powdered organic mix, to avoid the corn syrup that comes in the others, which I combine with a container of plain yogurt or Greek yogurt to make dips and spreads. Let's boost our immune systems by getting healthy probiotic nutrients from yogurt, used in place of the sour cream called for in dip recipes. You will not taste the difference! Our probiotic organisms are vulnerable critters; going in front of the firing squad each and every time we go on a course of antibiotics; we constantly need to replenish them. This is really important for those of you with Lyme Disease taking extended courses of antibiotics.

The beneficial bacteria in yogurt has already broken down the lactose sugar, which causes may people with lactose intolerance, pain and discomfort when eating or drinking dairy products. I eat yogurt daily to obtain the valuable bacteria we need for our immune system and colon health. Many of you have developed finicky GI systems as our illnesses progress; you might be able to introduce only *one teaspoon* of yogurt on the first day, slowly increasing the amount as your tolerance increases.

Greek yogurt, now hugely popular, has a much thicker texture and higher protein content than traditional yogurts. The fat is what gives it that wonderful, creamy consistency and the fat content often can be one-third of the product. This is saturated fat, so I stick to the organic brands such as *Stonyfield, Oikos* and *Maple Hill*.

The sour cream many people enjoy using on their baked potatoes, also contains helpful bacteria, most notably the organic brands that have added *lactobacillus acidophilus* and *bifidobacteria* cultures. These are the same two strains of bacteria that are commonly found in yogurts.

Not all brands of supermarket yogurt carry the same strains. *Stonyfield*, which I highly recommend, has six of them. For those of you with an interest in details, they are:

- Lactobacillus acidophilus
- Lactobacillus casei
- Lactobacillus reuteri
- Lactobacillus bifidus
- Lactobacillus bulgaricus and
- Streptococcus thermophilus.

Plain unsweetened yogurt is the best. You can add fruit or unsweetened fruit jam, to them, using honey as a sweetener. FAGE has a low sugar yogurt line called *Tru-Blend*. While not organic, they are part of the non-GMO project.

CHAPTER 9

THE BEVERAGE CART

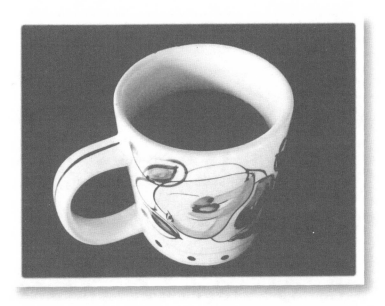

"As soon as coffee is in your stomach, there is a general commotion. Ideas begin to move...similes arise; the paper is covered. Coffee is your ally, and writing ceases to be a struggle."

~ Honore de Balzac (1779-1859)

There's nothing I enjoy more than holding a cup of pumpkin spice latte in my hand. I love to sip the aroma of cloves, cinnamon, and nutmeg in my coffee. Coffee has many health benefits, but there is also a downside for some of us. Many of us with chronic illness have difficulty tolerating caffeine. For me, the cut-off time is 3 p.m. Drinking a cup of caffeinated beverage after that time will cause me to lie awake all night, thinking about bills that are due, the leak in my roof, or the tree branches that need to be cut, instead of getting some shut-eye and dreaming of the day I win the Mega-millions draw. So, for me, coffee is best consumed at breakfast or mid-morning.

Some of my clients cannot tolerate any caffeine or suddenly they feel like they have been shot out of a cannon, unable to sit down or concentrate. There is a reason for this. Caffeine is a drug. The caffeine in coffee travels to our brain, increasing adrenaline, the stress hormone, and dopamine, the alertness hormone. Caffeine tolerance varies from one person to another. Though I'm not a big coffee drinker, I look forward to drinking flavored lattes during the holiday season. Research on the benefits of drinking coffee increases by the year. I have read that coffee drinker are less prone to developing *Parkinson's disease* and *Alzheimer's disease*, two very debilitating conditions that affect nerve transmission and brain function. Caffeine mobilizes fat from the body, so if you are able to exercise and want to lose weight, a cup of joe will assist you in burning the stores of fat around your belly. Those drinking coffee have a lower risk of two types of cancer: colorectal cancer is reduced 15%, and cancer of the liver, a much more deadly form of cancer, is reduced by 40%. However, we all know people who drink coffee and have these illnesses. Is it better to substitute other beverages? Here is what we do know about the downsides of caffeine. In some people, it causes rapid heartbeat, increases anxiety, and causes headaches, including the dreaded migraine. In addition, in women going through menopause, it can aggravate hot flashes, insomnia, and headaches. It can be a stomach irritant and cause frequent trips to the bathroom that may interfere with work. It can cause sleeplessness because it increases alertness hormones. In middle-aged to older adults, heavy coffee-drinking can leach the calcium from bones, setting you up for osteoporosis. Many of the studies finding health benefits from coffee are done with people drinking 4 to 5 cups a day. So what's a body to do? You really need to decide for yourself whether to continue consuming it. If you have acid reflux, hernia, or stomach ulcers, you probably want to reduce your intake of coffee. If you get migraines, you may want to reconsider your intake of caffeinated beverages. If you are a small-boned woman, you may want to add more milk to get some calcium with that coffee. Other beverages such as cola and tea also contain some caffeine. If you decide to lower your intake of caffeine, please do it GRADUALLY! I recommend keeping one cup of caffeinated beverage in the diet rather than cutting out all caffeine at once.

Cutting caffeine is not an easy thing to do. It needs to be withdrawn sneakily, so that you "trick" your body into not knowing that you are having less. We've all seen situation comedies with the characters that dropped coffee, cold-turkey, shaking uncontrollably, with blinding headaches, and bizarre brain symptoms. If you are drinking several cups of coffee in an attempt to stay awake, reduce one half a cup at a time until you are having just one cup of "Joe" in the morning because the stimulation in many cups of caffeine just overtaxes the adrenal glands.

Anyone with chronic illness, has *adrenal glands* working over-time. This is not often addressed in traditional medicine. Under ordinary circumstances, our adrenal glands, which sit one on top of each kidney, regulate, among many things, our blood sugar and the content of salt and water in our kidneys; they produce a small amount of sex hormone and create the hormone, *adrenaline*, which sounds just like the gland it comes from. Adrenaline is the hormone pouring through our bloodstream when we are wakened in the middle of the night from strange sounds in the house. As our heartbeats loudly throb in our chest, our breathing rates speed up, and we get sweaty palms as we reach for the baseball bat near the bed, to slay whatever monster has invaded our premises. Adrenaline is the same hormone that gives us superhuman strength to lift a heavy tree branch off the Porsche. It generates that quick burst of energy to either fight the enemy or flee the scene.

When we are sick, our adrenal glands use up vitamin C at an amazing rate and pour out adrenaline and another chemical called, *cortisol*, which fights infection. With the occurrence of Covid19, stress and the release of adrenaline finally received continued exposure in the news because one way to boost the immune system is to decrease the amount of stress you are placing on it. Even fighting chronic pain on a daily basis calls the adrenal gland into action with cortisol secreted to fight the threat. When the body perceives unending stress, eventually, a state of adrenal exhaustion sets in, with that gland barely getting a chance to rest. Therefore, it makes sense that we want to lessen the load on these vital glands.

Coffee beans, unfortunately, when grown conventionally, are sprayed with fungicides, herbicides, pesticides, and chemical fertilizers. It is best to purchase organic brands. In addition, to a difference in taste, organic coffee has a higher antioxidant profile.

This brings us back to caffeine; it raises heart rate and blood pressure and increases gut motility and alertness level. Remember, it increases your adrenal glands' production of adrenaline. So those poor adrenal glands are doing their job non-stop when you are drinking coffee throughout the day to stay awake. While traditional medicine does not address the adrenal gland function until 90% of it is lost, integrative and naturopathic doctors recommend a reduction in caffeine to their patients to give the adrenals a rest.

Unfortunately, for some people, removing all caffeine from the diet may cause more stress on the adrenal glands. So stick with one cup, if this works for you without driving you bonkers. If you are drinking coffee to be social or to keep warm, there are alternatives. I've never been a real coffee drinker and preferred tea. Now, I enjoy drinking hot water poured over a slice of fresh ginger to keep warm during the cold winter months. Ginger is a warming herb, and it also improves the digestive system. Drinking boiled water to which a bay leaf has also been added, aids in digestion with meals.

"Tea, tempers the spirit and harmonizes the mind, dispels lassitude and relieves fatigue, awakens thought and prevents drowsiness, lightens or refreshes the body, and clears the perceptive faculties."
~ Confucius

ARE WE DOING AS CONFUCIUS SAYS?

People in the U.S. are rather closely divided on drinking coffee or tea, with 54% of the population drinking coffee daily, and the remaining 46% drinking tea. The favored tea is black and strong, echoing Confucius's comments about "awakening thought." There are many hot beverages available containing less caffeine than coffee. Teas are now available in so many varieties; take a look at the tea section in your supermarket. They practically take up the entire aisle these days. You can find red, (Roobis), naturally caffeine-free, white, green, and black. Three of them, black, white, and green, are grown from the same plant—*camellia sinensis*. The type of processing they undergo after they are picked determines the amount of health-boosting polyphenols they contain. All of them contain catechins, *flavonoids* and *polyphenols*. Let's take a closer look at the main ones.

WHITE TEA

The making of white tea is relatively simple, requiring very little processing. The tea plant's silvery-white buds are picked before they open, making for the least bitter tea. The young leaves are sun-dried or rapidly steamed and dried. Because they undergo no fermentation process, the tea leaves contain three times the antioxidant activity of either green or black. Researchers at Oregon State University studied white tea for its ability to kill lymphoma and leukemia in mice by putting the extracts of lemon grass and white tea extract in their drinking water.[34] Now we wait until research shows promise that white tea may act the same in humans.

GREEN TEA

There is little processing needed to make green tea, with its properties of boosting the immune system and assisting weight loss. Green tea contains a specific polyphenol called *catechin* with natural anti-fungal properties. After the tea leaves are picked, they are allowed to wither and die, then fried in an oven or pan for quick dehydrating. They can also be steamed or parched. The final step is rolling them. As a result of these relatively "gentle" heating methods, green tea catechins, flavonoids, and polyphenols do not

---

[34] Philion, C., Ma, D., Ruvinov, I., Mansour, F., Pignanelli, C., Noel, M.,...& Pandy, S. (2017) Cymbopogon citratus and camellia sinensis extracts selectively induce apoptosis in cancer cells and reduce growth of lymphoma xenografts in vivo. *Oncotarget, 8(67), 110756*

undergo destruction that happens in the making of black tea, nor do the leaves undergo any fermentation. As a result, many healthy substances such as EGCG or *epigallocatechin gallate*, are still abundant, and the flavonoid, theaflavin, is preserved. You have probably seen advertisements on TV and on the net for EGCG as a weight loss supplement. This compound boosts the metabolism making food calories burn more efficiently and can be found in several weight loss aids. Many people boil the water regardless of what type of tea they prepare. However, with green tea, it's not necessary to boil the water. Green tea can actually become bitter when steeped at the high temperatures that black tea bags require. So, if you tried green tea in the past, not realizing this, and brought the water to a boil, you may like to try it again.

Research on people with the chronic liver disease, NAFLD or *non-alcoholic fatty liver disease* shows some promise for those with this liver's inflammation, which has many causes, including viruses and toxin exposure. Using green tea extracts has been successful. However, research also shows liver damage resulting from using high dosages of EGCG. This is an example of the whole food being superior to an extract. In a study of Chinese men and women, those who drank green tea for long periods of time, 20 years or more, were protected against developing liver cancer. Green tea may also be beneficial for our heart health. The *catechins* in green tea prevent blood clots, inflammation of the blood vessels, and improve the vessels' ability to dilate[35] so that more blood can flow through them. This is excellent news for those with a family history of high blood pressure. But as it is with all things, you never want

---

[35] Xu, R., Yang, K., Ding, J., & Chen, G. (2010). Effect of green tea supplementation on blood pressure: A systematic review and meta-analysis of randomized controlled trials. *Medicine* Feb 2020 Vol 99 (6) doi:10.1097/MD.0000000000019047

to over-do it; don't go about drinking more than six cups of green tea per day.

BLACK TEA

Are you staring into a cup of black tea as you read this book? Our daughters have tea parties imitating us with their stuffed animals and dolls. Women host tea parties where tea is served with pastries, especially in the UK where mid-afternoon is dedicated as "tea time." There are also reams of information about black tea because it has been such a popular beverage for centuries. Many people drink it because it contains less caffeine, 50 milligrams than the 60-175 found in a coffee cup. Black tea may help to offset the side-effects of drowsiness and lethargy that can occur from pain medications without that caffeine jolt you get from coffee. However, the journey from the tea in your cup to its origin in the plant requires the greatest amount of processing. The leaves are picked, and they sit out in the sun to oxidize or ferment, which gives them their flavor. Then they are steamed. However, the heating processes destroy more specific antioxidants called *anthocyanins*, commonly found in red or blue foods such as strawberries and blueberries. Black tea also contains phenol compounds and tannins. Do you know how your mouth and tongue feel dry when you drink tea? Tannins give it that astringent property.

Research is underway to discover the relationship between bone density and black tea consumption. In one study of men and women from Taiwan who drank tea, bone mineral density was found to be consistently higher than in non-tea drinkers.[36] The bone's protection could be from the fluoride found naturally in tea leaves or from the phyto-estrogen effects that tea contains. Caution is advised about drinking more than 5 cups of black tea, as it may exaggerate many medications' effects. Pregnant women should not have more than 2 cups of black tea per day.

RED TEA

How many of you are familiar with red tea? Not very high in tannins compared to the green, white, and black varieties, red tea originates from a different plant. Its scientific name is *aspalathus linearis* and it has grown for greater than 300 years in South Africa. Red tea contains unique antioxidants, *rutin* and *quercetin*, both beneficial for our immune systems, as well as orientin. *Roobis* red tea has been used for centuries overseas to cure infantile colic, and as a cough expectorant. Lately, the focus in the United States is on using it to prevent wrinkles. Because it has fewer of the bitter tannins found in black tea; Roobis Red tea has a milder flavor.

HERBAL TEAS

Your supermarket is filled with herbal teas creating tasty variations on black and green teas. Fruit extracts are dried and then combined in tea bags to make blueberry tea, cranberry, spiced apple, lemon, or honey vanilla. If you are watching the amount of caffeine you consume, be sure to check the label. Some herbal teas also contain black tea combined with the fruit. *Chamomile* is a caffeine-free tea,

---

[36] Wu, C.H., Yao, W.J., Lu, F.H., Wu, J.S., & Chang, C.J. (2002). Epidemiological Evidence of Increased Bone Mineral Density in Habitual Tea Drinkers. *Archives of internal Medicine*,162(9), 1001-1006 http://doi:10.1001/archinte.162.9.1001

very relaxing, and is often combined with mint leaves. I enjoy drinking chamomile with supper. When you choose an herbal tea, read the label carefully to account for all the ingredients used. This is particularly important if you have either allergies or high blood pressure. Ingredients such as Ginseng and Rhodiola will make the blood pressure rise, which could be dangerous for some people. Those with certain environmental allergies, such as pollen, could experience a cross-reaction with chamomile. Ginger tea makes a gentle digestive aid and is often sold during the Holidays.

WHAT ABOUT THE DECAF BEVERAGES?

Decaffeinated coffees and teas can create more work for our livers to process them, as the chemicals used in removing the caffeine can be harmful to those already struggling with immune system problems. I prefer to have one cup of caffeinated tea then drink other beverages throughout the day rather than abstaining from all caffeine.

I remember my stay fondly with friends on an organic farm. I used to wander into the kitchen, still sleepy-eyed, inhaling the delicious aroma of an herbal beverage that resembles coffee. This hot drink permeating the house with its aroma is called *Cafix*, and is made from barley, chicory, and malt. *Pero*, made from barley, chicory, and rye, is another one that is totally caffeine-free and tastes similar to instant coffee. Then there is *Teeccino* which has carob in it and considered the sweetest. Of course, for those looking for something to help you focus yet remain calm, you can turn to *Ayurvedic Roast*, which I have never personally tried, but it came up on a google search of the six best tasting coffee substitutes.

In addition to coffee and teas, there is hot cocoa. If chocolate is your drug of choice as it is mine, purchase organic hot cocoa mix, free of Trans fats and corn syrup. Corn syrup is not a good sweetener. It is loaded with pesticide residue and a proven cause of obesity. Unfortunately, the American corn supply is in jeopardy due to the genetic manipulation of the crop as well as the competition to use it as fuel for cars.

THE DANGER OF ARTIFICIAL SWEETENERS

I steer away from cocoa mixes containing artificial sugars and artificial sweeteners, which are suspected *carcinogens* and proven to have adverse effects on the brain in some people. Artificial sugars are also a threat to your waistline, as they do not create the insulin response our bodies have to sugar and can trick the brain into consuming more. The artificial sweeteners as a group are bad news, causing obesity, conditions of being overweight, type 2 diabetes, and metabolic syndrome.[37] A multi-ethnic study of adults across the country, was carried out between 2002 to 2007 on the effects of drinking sodas containing artificial sweeteners daily. The results were pretty striking, with people having a 36% higher risk of metabolic syndrome and a 67% rate of having Type 2 Diabetes.[38] Now, as to other artificial sweeteners, a study done in China from Harbin Medical University on mice reported, "The constant use of food additives such as sucralose and saccharin may be more

---

[37] Swithers, S.E. (2013). Artificial sweeteners produce the counterintuitive effect of inducing metabolic derangements. *Trends in Endocrinology & Metabolism*, 24(9), 431-441

[38] Nettleton, J.A., Lutsey, P.L., Wang, Y., Lima, J.A., Michos, E.D., & Jacobs, D.R. (2009). Diet Soda intake and risk of Incident metabolic syndrome and type 2 diabetes in the multi-ethnic study of atherosclerosis (MESA). *Diabetes Care*, 32(4) 688-694 http://doi.org/10.2337/dc08-1799

detrimental to gut microbiota and health than antibiotics."[39] They fed mice sucralose, and they developed colorectal tumors. Many of you reading this have been diagnosed with IBD, or Inflammatory Bowel Disease. These can range from Colitis to Crohn's Disease and are being diagnosed in young adults and children! According to Dr. Xiaota Qin, "IBD has become one of the most common chronic inflammatory conditions only after Rheumatoid arthritis with millions of patients around the world."[40] He combed over the literature around the world and, when aspartame was introduced, he noticed significant increases in IBD in countries that approved its use, including Canada and the United States. When sucralose hit the market, he noticed a similar spike in IBD cases. His theory is that sucralose impairs the bacteria that we need for a healthy intestine, and then inactivates the enzymes needed to digest food resulting in a destruction of the protective mucous layer. Then inflammation sets in, and undigested food particles are able to set up more inflammation with food intolerances. The problem begins to extend beyond our digestive systems with inflammation of the joints, skin, eyes, and mouth.

How many of you suffer headaches or, worse, migraines? Have you ever considered the possibility? Could it be the artificial sweetener you are using? I had a client come to me for help with her headaches, and she told me that she never used any artificial sweeteners- ever. Turns out the stick of chewing gum she had in her purse was filled with aspartame. Known to many of us as Nutra Sweet, or Equal, aspartame goes by other names you may see on restaurant packets of sweetener called Sugar Twin and Amino

---

[39] Li, X., Liu, Y., Wang, Y., Li, X., Guo, M., & Jiang, M. (2020). Sucralose promotes colitis-associated colorectal cancer risk in a murine model along with changes in microbiota. *Frontiers in Oncology* 10, 710 http://doi/10.3389/fonc.2020.00710

[40] Qin, X. (2012). Etiology of inflammatory bowel disease: a unified hypotheses. *World journal of Gastroenterology* WJG,18(15), 1708

Sweet. They are all composed of the same two amino acids: *phenylalanine* and *aspartic acid* with a methyl ester. The methyl portion of the chemical causes problems as it turns into methanol in our bodies. You remember that during the first wave of Covid19, some of the hand sanitizers had to be recalled because they were made of Methanol, wood alcohol, rather than ethanol or drinking alcohol. Methanol is poison to the human body, and it turns into formaldehyde. If you have children, please look over the labels of the cough medicines that your child uses. They are often made with aspartame and if anyone of any age gets those Kool-Aid drink packs, beware. They contain sucralose.

SWEET ENOUGH?

As if our adrenal glands didn't have enough drama, with the secretion of glucocorticoid and cortisol production to counteract inflammation, along comes table sugar or *sucrose* which makes them work even harder. Table sugar, sucrose, is a refined white sugar and the unpleasant news about it, continues to increase. I will start with the risk of Heart Disease. A study was published in Circulation[41] analyzing the results of the Health professional follow up study. Their focus was on 42, 883 Doctors given surveys of the beverages they drank. Those drinking beverages that contained sugar had a 20% higher risk of heart attacks than those drinking "diet" beverages. The men who were drinking sugar-sweetened beverages also had higher triglycerides, more inflammation markers (C-reactive protein), tumor necrosis factor, and

---

[41] de Koning, L., Malik, V.S., Kellogg, M.D., Rimm, E.B., Willett, W.C., & Hu, F.B. (2018) Sweetened beverage consumption, incident coronary heart disease, and biomarkers of risk in men. *Circulation* 125(14), 1735-1741. doi.org/10.1161/CIRCULATIONAHA.111.067017

Interluekin-6. They also had lower levels of the good HDL that we all want to have.

Now let's look at a study on women. The Nurses Health Study looked at women to determine the relationship between drinking sugar-sweetened beverages with the risk of Heart attack and found similar findings. The 88, 520 women were nurses ages 30-55. Those who habitually drank sugar-sweetened beverages, had lower levels of the good cholesterol, HDL, and higher levels of the marker for inflammation, C-reactive protein.[42]

The truth is that sugar, also referred to as sucrose, affects our gut microbiome's composition; those billions of bacteria that maintain our health. Some bacteria help in the creation of B vitamins and others that are associated with our immune health. Therefore, we don't want to mess around with them and destroy the balance. An altered gut microbiome is associated with IBS, gas and bloating, behavior problems in children. It alters our hormones, contributes to joint inflammation, and worst of all, it ruins the skin. You have seen advertisements for *collagen*, a component of our skin. Sugar attaches to collagen and ages the skin by creating A.G.E.S. (Advanced Glycation End products). These further destroy the latticework that collagen creates for skin structure and elastin found in the skin, causing wrinkles. The horror, right?

Sugar also impairs hormone levels by causing insulin resistance over time. The hormone insulin, has the job of carrying the sugar we eat into the cells of our bodies. It can be used in two ways; we burn it to get the energy to take that golf swing. Or we store it as

---

[42] Yu, Z., Ley, S.H., Sun, Q., Hu, F.B., & Malik, V.S. (2018). Cross-sectional association between sugar-sweetened beverage intake and cardiometabolic biomarkers in U.S. women. *British Journal of Nutrition,* 119(5), 570-580. DOI: https://doi.org/10.1017/s00071145170003841

fat. In addition, this fat is metabolically active, creating its own hormones, which can lead to obesity and other illness.

Also, Sugar has an impact on Diabetes. In a review by Swedish researchers on the study of sugar, they found high sugar consumption, has an impact on the development of type 2 Diabetes. When they looked at people consuming 2 or more sugar-containing beverages per week, (there can be 13 tsp. of sugar in a 12-ounce serving of soda), there was a "relatively consistent association of sugar-sweetened beverages with Type 2 Diabetes."[43]

Sucrose makes our livers work hard to break it down to a more usable form called glucose. At Johns Hopkins University, mice were fed sucrose and developed inflamed livers. I made the switch to using honey in my tea. Unprocessed stevia with zero calories, used in other countries for over 7 centuries, is another popular choice. Because Stevia is so sweet, very little of it is needed.

Let's summarize that artificial sweeteners cause metabolic problems and increase risk of stroke and heart disease, and sucrose also increases the risk of heart attacks and Diabetes. What are we to do? I recommend that we consume sugar-sweetened beverages diluted with seltzer water or tonic water if you want a different flavor. When I'm having tea, I remove the tea bag before it becomes bitter and requires a sweetener. For those times when I'm craving sugar, I put raw honey, full of probiotics, into my tea, and raw honey doesn't cause the disruption in the gut biome that sugar does.

---

[43] Sonestedt, E., Øverby, N., Laaksonen, D., & Eva Birgisdottir, B. (2012). Does high sugar consumption exacerbate cardiometabolic risk factors and increase the risk of type 2 diabetes and cardiovascular disease? Food and Nutrition Research, 56(1), 19014.
ncbi.nim.nih.gov/pmc/articles/PMC3409338/doi: 10.3402/fnr.v56i0.19104

AGAVE NECTAR AND HONEY

My favorite sweetener has to be raw blue agave nectar. No, it is not blue. It's a colorless syrup, which comes from a cactus plant growing in the Southwest. Raw Agave, not to be confused with processed agave, that you find in the supermarket these days, has the same 16 calories per teaspoon as table sugar but tends not to cause the surges in blood sugar associated with table sugar. Remember, the job of insulin from the pancreas is to remove sugar from the blood stream to get it into our hungry cells. Many of us with chronic illness, maybe from inadequate nutrition before we got sick, the inability to exercise, or the stress of coping with chronic pain, are at greater risk of developing a condition called *insulin resistance*. Unprocessed, raw agave will not cause any insulin resistance problems that can occur with processed agave.

Insulin resistance is bad news. It basically means that our cells partially closed the door to sugar so that more insulin is required to push it in through the membrane. This happens over a while from eating too much sugar and refined carbohydrates. Obesity and inactivity also contribute to this state, but obesity can also be a *result* from insulin resistance. With the use of minimally processed raw agave or honey, you won't trigger as much of an insulin response. Both are easy to use for sweetening tea, drizzling over cereal, and can be used to bake whole grain waffles, pancakes, and other goodies when you get your energy back.

COLD BEVERAGES

NOT ALL JUICES ARE HIGH IN SUGAR

Sometimes, a cold beverage is what you are thirsting for, especially when the weather is warm. Unsweetened iced tea, black or green, makes a healthy refreshing choice that is easy to prepare. Just add ice cubes to the tea you steeped earlier. The supermarkets are brimming with prepared iced teas, but you need to be a discriminating consumer because some brands are full of corn syrup, which we should step aside from as a sweetener. The organic brands offer unsweetened, sweetened with honey, agave, or stevia. What about juices? Some juice choices can be counted as a serving of fruit, but we need to remember that juice is high in sugar content. Apple, grape, and cranberry juices, because they contain nutrients from the flesh of the fruit as well as the skins, offer more nutritional value. However, rather than drinking them full strength, I pour filtered drinking water into a glass, leaving one inch from the top, then add just a splash of cranberry or grape juice. Sipped throughout the day, I know I can enjoy drinking juice without causing surges of insulin.

Did you know that cloudy apple juice is higher in antioxidant activity than clear, even though cloudy doesn't look quite as appealing? Fall harvest season is not the only time to enjoy apple and cranberry juices and cranberry has a unique property. Unsweetened cranberry juice can act as a car wash for the bladder. It not only cleanses the urinary tract but keeps bacteria from sticking to the bladder walls.

The compounds in unsweetened cranberry juice when taken full strength, contain measurable amounts of *quercetin* and *myricetin*, which prevent sticky plaque from adhering to our teeth.[44]

Grape juice is a good source of resveratrol that ups the metabolism and protects the heart but is very high in sugar. Notice how it is syrupy thick? So I combine it with a less sweet ne such as Pomegranate. This makes a tasty drink and cuts the amount of sugar entering the bloodstream at one interval. Pomegranate juice has so many antioxidants that protect our earts!

Last, but important, is orange juice. A glass of orange juice provides the DRI for vitamin C and is full of potassium. For those who experience heartburn from drinking OJ in the morning, try having it with lunch or a snack. You may find it less likely to irritate those delicate membranes of the mouth and GI tract or, once again, dilute it with seltzer water or tonic water. As long as you don't have high blood pressure, the tonic water's added salt should not cause a rise in blood pressure.

KEEPING OUR DIETS STRAIGHT

Sometimes a vegetable-based beverage will hit the spot. I enjoy drinking vegetable and tomato juices. Bolthouse Farms distributes a tasty vegetable juice. I also enjoy V8 juice when I need salt. A 12 oz. bottle of V8 supplies us with two servings of vegetables. Suppose you have been diagnosed with *candida*, you may have been advised to avoid drinking fruit juices because the natural sugar in them, feeds the organisms that are over-populated in this

---

[44] Duarte, S., Gregoire, S., Singh, A.P., Vorsa, N., Schaich, K., Bowen, W.H., & Koo, H. Inhibitory effects of cranberry polyphenols on formation of streptococcus mutans biofilms. *FEMS Microbiology Letters*, (2006) 257(1), 50-56. http://doi.org/10.1111/j.1574-6968.2006.00147

yeast overgrowth condition. The least processed vegetable juices you can find, such as celery, carrot, or tomato, will make great options while you are abstaining from the fruity beverages.

STRUCK DOWN!

How many out there enjoy drinking soda? You may have noticed the soda bottles and cans becoming smaller as researchers make the ominous link of the consumption of sugary sodas with obesity and diabetes. It's not easy to give up a habit that you may have enjoyed for decades. Fortunately, healthy alternatives will make you feel like you are drinking those sugary soft drinks but won't contain the harmful phosphates that compete for calcium absorption in our bones.

If not filled with sugar and corn syrup, sodas are filled with unnatural sweeteners like Aspartame, Sucralose, Splenda, and Acesulfame K. Anyone with chronic health problems is best advised to avoid all these sweeteners. These require too much processing by the liver, which is already overwhelmed by the need to break down all the pills, capsules, and other potions that we use for control over our illness every day. In addition, the phosphorous in soda leaches calcium from our bones and sodas because of their sugar content, lower the potassium in our blood needed for healthy muscle contraction and relaxation. Have you ever experienced a Charley horse? This gripping pain can be very intense! Anyone who has ever experienced one is not likely to forget it. Potassium, along with calcium and magnesium, is needed to prevent cramps.

Carbonated beverages can still be worked into our eating plans by switching to natural sodas that are made the old-fashioned way. They have fewer ingredients: no corn syrup, just sugar. Of course, you don't want to drink these daily. Remember a Swedish research that found just two servings of sugar-sweetened beverages was associated with diabetes? So reserve them for special occasions, perhaps one day of the weekend. Chinese ginger soda is one I enjoy occasionally, and *Reeds Real Ginger Ale and Bruce Cost Ginger Ale* are made of only 4 ingredients. Both are available on Amazon. Have you tried any of the sparkling waters, such as *"The Switch Orange Tangerine,"* made up of 100% juice? *Izze Sparkling* Blueberry, Pomegranate, or Grapefruit with their refreshing clean flavors? They also are made from 100% fruit juice. Look for sparkling water that has flavor but no sweeteners and combine it with 100% fruit juice.

There are neither phosphates, preservatives, nor artificial dyes in any of the natural sodas. Some other cold beverages you might reserve for special occasions are fruit juice-tea combinations. Some use red and others use green tea. It's another way to get a good supply of antioxidants. Just check the label to be sure that what you purchase is sweetened with fruit juice, rather than added sucrose. Those that list "corn syrup" on the label are not going to enhance anyone's immune system nor are those containing artificial sweeteners. The fruit-juice sweetened teas have enough sweetness for my taste buds and I really appreciate that they come in glass bottles rather than plastic. Some plastics, as you are aware, contain harmful chemicals, like BPA, which has been linked to a host of health problems, including cancer development.

CHAPTER 10

MAKING MEALS WORK FOR YOU!

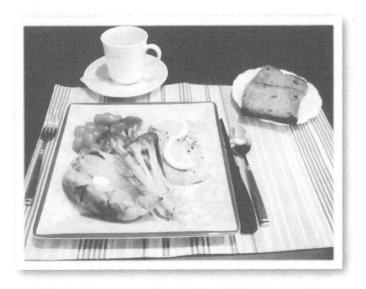

ROASTING + DELI FOOD = MEAL!

O kay, today is a bad day. You managed to get through breakfast then needed to return to bed. It's convenient to have a pork roast in the freezer for days like these when you may have awakened to the feeling that a big rig ran you over. You can defrost the pork in the refrigerator while you rest, have it ready to cook by suppertime, and have many more meals to come from that simple step. See my roast pork idea.

Does the idea of roasting any meat send shivers up your spine? Do you conjure up images of that night when you first cooked supper for the in-laws? I know you forgot to remove the giblets in that little plastic bag and cooked the bird with the bag inside. Your mashed potatoes were lumpy, and all of your vegetables turned to brown mush while you tried to rescue the potatoes. Put all of that behind you. Roasting a pork sounds like a great deal of work, but it's deceptively simple. (Look at my simple recipe)

ROAST PORK LOIN

- o 1 lb. pork tenderloin
- o 1-2 cloves of garlic
- o 2 Tbsp. orange marmalade

1. Set the oven to 425°F.
2. Line the cookie sheet or roasting pan with aluminum foil or parchment paper
3. Crush the clove(s) garlic and slather it all over the pork tenderloin
4. Add marmalade
5. Place pork into heated oven, inserting an oven thermometer into thickest portion.
6. Set timer for 30 minutes

When pork reaches 150 degrees on the thermometer, it's ready to be sliced and served!

Roasting chicken isn't that much harder. There's one extra step involved, rinsing the chicken parts first, under the kitchen faucet, before placing them in a pan. Fill the pan with more clean water, not the rinse water. After taking it from the water and patting it dry with a paper towel, just add a dusting of your dry spice rub or a dash of ground black pepper before baking it in the oven. Baking and roasting are pretty much the same thing. It's also convenient to add a side-serving of grains such as soba noodles from the salad bar or tabouleh from the deli case. The grain dishes go well with sweet cranberry chutney, which comes in a jar. Did you know that cranberries also contain those all-important antioxidants? This time it's lutein and zeaxanthin, just like kiwifruit, which can protect against some forms of cancer.

By munching on some pre-cut celery or carrot sticks or adding a few marinated artichokes to your dinner plate, you can boost the nutrients in that meal or rely on good lettuce. If you haven't already had one today, open a package of fresh organic blends of lettuce. I enjoy Olivia's Organics, Asian, or herb mix. These salads come pre-washed in convenient clamshell packages and supply you with those all-important leafy greens, full of electrolytes and antioxidants and flavor!

Other quick and simple meals can be crafted from pre-made salads such as the chickpea, black bean, or lentil Mediterranean salads sold in the produce area. Cedars has done all the work for you with their delicious lentil salad, loaded with lentils, crunchy red peppers, bathed in olive oil, and dotted with carrots. I serve this on a bed of lettuce, alongside a prepared soup such as carrot-ginger, velvety butternut squash, or a rich tomato, all of which are brimming in antioxidants and pleasing to the palate.

Some delis sell falafel patties, made from ground chickpea parties fashioned into a tasty burger shape. These are great, crumbled on top of salads, or you can eat them between two hearty slices of sourdough or sprouted bread. Sprouted breads are not in the category of white bread People who are intolerant to wheat can often better tolerate sprouted breads.

> **NOTE:** Wheat intolerance is not to be confused with gluten intolerance or Celiac disease, which is a serious illness.

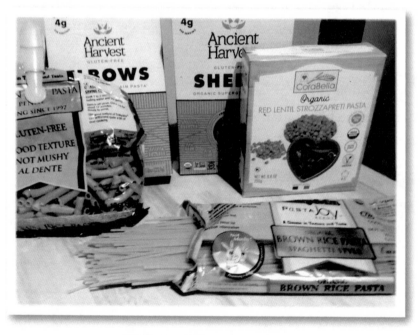

IT'S PASTA NIGHT!

Growing up in an Irish-Italian family, one side was destined to take over. Since my Italian grandmother lived with us and did the cooking until she was 80 years old, guess which side came to predominate? This is where my love of all things pasta comes from.

Growing up with my Nana, when we were down with fever, she would prepare pastina cooked in water with a teaspoon of butter. Sometimes she would add an egg for some extra protein. I looked forward to having those tiny little balls of semolina, sliding down my throat as a child, and I continue to relish this when having a stressful day. It's easy to prepare when I walk in the door. A while later, when I am feeling better, I sauté some green vegetables and snack on fruit.

Now I've expanded my supply of pasta dishes to include those made from brown rice, quinoa, rice and millet combined, bean flour, and occasionally wheat. Brown rice pasta is so easy to cook, tasty, and just as nutritious as whole-wheat pasta, as it supplies 3 grams fiber per serving, the same as the bean ones. I know it sounds strange: pasta made from beans? Just 3/4 cup of red lentil pasta supplies 4 grams of fiber! If we are trying to reach the government recommendations for 38 grams for fiber for men, and 25 for women. (The number of grams drops slightly for men and women over age 50, to 30 and 21 respectively), we need to be build fiber into every meal and snack. In addition, they come in an increasing variety of shapes. Corn pasta is available in elbow, spaghetti, rotini, and small shells. Only buy organic corn pasta because conventional corn in this country is genetically modified. We don't want to be guinea pigs in a huge experiment of the population eating GMO food. Rice pasta is available in long strands of spaghetti or wider fettuccini, elbows, penne, rotini, and even in Lasagna strips and large shells to use for stuffing. Two of my favorite toppings are robust tomato marinara sauce and fresh basil and pesto. Pesto sauce originally was ground parsley with pine nuts and flavored with garlic. Now all kinds of pesto can be found, created out of nuts and other veggies. Try the arugula one sometime to get the benefits of broccoli and cauliflower from a crucifer that has no semblance to either, yet gives us those sulfur-containing substances we need for our detoxification pathways.

Popular with so many, pasta meals can be very healthy and it doesn't make you overweight at all for those of you watching your waistline. Just add more fiber, and that's a cinch to do by adding frozen vegetables. Just add the veggies during the last five minutes of cooking to avoid over-cooking. Next, strain the pasta and vegetables together and add a flavorful tomato-based sauce. Whole wheat pasta has fiber in it that you won't find in traditional pasta but early on in my nutrition program, when the focus is on making your GI tract feel less irritable, I ask you to choose whole wheat less often. Try a pasta made from a grain other than wheat. Corn, quinoa, and rice pasta are just as versatile as the wheat variety, and some cook more quickly than wheat. They come in dried forms at present. Quinoa pasta contains more protein per serving, which is important for those whose muscles are not getting much exercise or are losing muscle due to illness and/or disuse. Also, the bean pasta provides us with 14 grams of protein, twice that of regular wheat pasta. Spelt and Kamut Pasta are available, darker in color than what you expect pasta to be, but served with a robust sauce or an Italian vinaigrette as a pasta salad; these offer you two more options that taste great.

Dried pasta has the advantage of sitting on the shelf for a few months. The gluten-free pasta make life much easier for those of us with wheat intolerance. Wheat intolerance is on the rise in this country. Some of the wheat in the United States, has been altered genetically to make it more pest-resistant. This involves inserting actual pesticides into the genetic structure of the seeds. The bigger picture then is the wheat we are eating today is not the same as the wheat that your grandmother and great grandmother ate in their day. Wheat today, actually has extra gluten added to it, which may be responsible for increasing GI trouble, rapidly increasing in young people.

Pasta meals cannot be surpassed for convenience. Regular Pasta takes approximately 12 minutes to cook on the stove, and the others cook even faster. I'm not recommending you stand at the counter chopping up carrots and peppers here. We're just opening a jar of sauce and pouring it over the cooked pasta. Let's increase the nutritional value by cutting open a poly bag of red peppers, fresh sliced mushrooms, a jar of sliced artichokes, or a can of cooked black beans. (These give us vitamins and minerals, increase the fiber content of the meal, and taste good!). Then add the red sauce. Now you've created a more robust meal without adding many calories, not expending much sweat, and it's full of nutrients to swat away those free radicals in our body that accumulate every time we breathe.

Ramen noodles are very convenient, and when I wrote my first draft, I was pretty much all over them, and I still tell everyone to stay away from the commercially packaged ones —the curly ones with the salty flavoring-pack. They contain 14 grams of fat in one block, and are fried, also loaded with trans-fat and hydrogenated oil as well as MSG, which hides under other names. However, organic ramen noodles are now available! Look for KOYO brand Ramen organic noodles made with heirloom grains and vegan. They also contain that little paper packet of flavorings, but these have only 1 gram of fat. These also have the non-GMO verified seal on them. They supply 2 grams of fiber! and 7 grams of protein! I have them occasionally and always add a serving of veggies to them, usually frozen peas, organic corn, or canned mushrooms. Because they contain no preservatives, I even put them into my food program in this book! There are nourishing options for instant meals you will find in the healthy section of your supermarket. Look for Dr. McDougall's, which actually provide anywhere from 8 to 21 grams of protein per serving depending on what you purchase. You can find instant split pea soup, black bean, pad Thai and Asian noodle instant cups. Both of these are supplied in paper cups for extra convenience, so you can bring them to work, pour in some boiled water and eat some raw vegetables to cover the nutrients for this meal.

Are you looking for grains that cook quickly while offering the convenience of pasta? Choose rice cellophane noodles, soba noodles, quick-cooking barley, and couscous. Rice cellophane noodles barely need any cooking but do need to soak—for five minutes. Then you lower them into boiling water for perhaps one or two minutes. Cellophane noodles are not made from a grain, but from mung bean flour but do not taste like beans in any way, I assure you. Soba noodles, made of 100% buckwheat, are great for those who want to lessen the burden on your stomach and intestines. You won't find them in a box; They come in small bundles, about six in a cellophane package. Make sure you read the ingredient label, because noodles sold as "buckwheat," are not always 100% buckwheat and might contain wheat.

Here's an idea: Instead of standing to chop herbs on a cutting board you can use my method. I simply tear arugula leaves or snip them with scissors and add them to the sauce towards the very end of the cooking time, so everything heats together in one savory pot. Anyone who truly hates broccoli out there will be very pleased to know that arugula is in the crucifer family with it but has nowhere near the same taste! It's rich in antioxidants, special ones with very long names, *iso-thio-cyanates*. These prevent cancer by interfering with the signals used in a pathway that would create tumors. Other nutrient boosters are the fresh shiitake mushrooms, full of natural killer cell boosters I add to my sauces and salads. Who doesn't need that extra help?

When it is a chore just to get your socks on, you want yourself surrounded by ready-to-eat but nutritious foods. This is a high priority of mine to always have nutrient-dense foods available in the house, those with the highest antioxidant profile, compared to calories. Remember the charts of fruits and vegetables I supplied back in chapter 7, the Fighter Nutrients? My body literally craves the electrolytes in these, and when I don't eat enough, my mouth becomes dry in a way that water will not correct. Then there is the fiber content of the produce.

Dietary fiber becomes even more important when we are not able to climb Mount Koji or go wind-surfing in Oahu. Adding to this, constipation, is often a dreaded side effect of the medications you may be taking for pain, spasms, depression, anxiety, and sleep. Some of you reading this may be suffering from IBS or irritable bowel syndrome. This condition is poorly understood by traditional medicine. In addition to a poorly balanced micro-biome, the environment of microbes in our intestines; many cases are due to undiagnosed food intolerances, and are now linked to many of the auto-immune diseases as well. A nutritionist communicating with your physician can give you an elimination diet and a food challenge to find out to what foods you are reacting to.

Have you ever had one of those days when you needed to have macaroni and cheese for your SANITY? We all have them, especially those of us with restrictions on our gluten consumption. There's something about being told that you need to avoid a food that conjures up intense cravings, and even maybe dreams about the foods when you finally hit the sack that night, even when it wasn't your absolute favorite to begin with. It's as though the emotional center of the brain, the amygdala, became rewired so that all the receptors for the foods you're supposed to eat suddenly become boring and unappealing, and the receptors for the "forbidden" foods seem to multiply tenfold and light up your brain cells like a Las Vegas Strip at night. They lure you down that aisle where they're located, practically calling you by name!

Good news! There is a delicious frozen gluten-free macaroni and cheese entree called Amy's rice macaroni and cheese waiting in your grocer's freezer case. You will get a portion size that will be appropriate. Those of you with chronic stomach grumbles, may just find this one more digestible. Moreover, for those of you who are dairy-free, there is a dairy-free version as well. The pasta is made of rice instead of wheat, and the entire dinner is completely gluten-free and, may I add—delicious! To compensate for the high fat content of comfort foods like this—it's the FAT, that we are craving—after it cooks, just mix in one cup of your favorite frozen vegetables, heated in a small amount of water while the mac cooks in the oven. My favorite is turnip greens. The cheese sauce not only complements the greens but by combining the two, you get 36% of your day's need for Calcium. That's great for our bones and muscles. The greens also supply us with one-quarter of our daily vitamin A allotment; the vitamin that feeds our skin and our immune systems. All those retinoid and retinol anti-wrinkle formulations you find on the market are derivatives of this vitamin.

MORE GOOD NEWS

The turnips and greens have zero fat, zero cholesterol, 2 valuable grams of fiber, and you are getting potassium, which offsets some of the sodium found in the macaroni and cheese. So enjoy—but not too often.

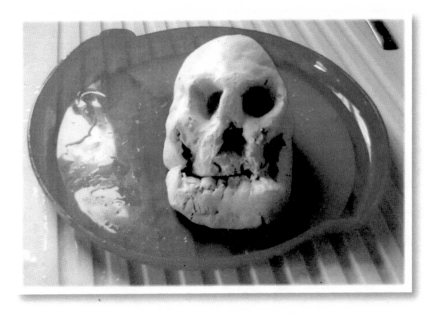

CHAPTER 11

FOOD ALLERGIES AND INTOLERANCES

HOLD THE VEAL!

Here you are, sitting in your favorite Italian restaurant-the aroma of garlic and basil perfumes the air. Hung on the walls are colorful paintings of Venice with its graceful gondolas floating along the canals. A magnum of vino and plastic grapes decorates the corners. A tarantella may be playing in the background. You are seated at a table covered with a red and white checkered tablecloth and holding one of those menus with the leather cover.

The Veal Parmigiana looks tempting tonight, so you ask the waiter (since you have an allergy to peanuts) if there is any peanut oil used in the sauce. The waiter is not aware that a new chef is substituting tonight, who does not use pure olive oil in the sauce. Here comes the piping hot entree. You dig into it with your fork. Oh-oh! You feel tingling on your tongue and lips. Realizing that someone in the kitchen was ignorant tonight, you make a dash into the rest room to use your portable epinephrine device to buy you some time before the swelling spreads from your tongue to your airways. In this case, you get to the ER on time, to receive life-saving treatment.

This is how it used to be for millions of people before a law was passed in many states that restaurants need to address food allergies. Every place serving food must have a sign posted for customers to see, informing you, the customer—if you have any food allergies—to inform the staff know about it because they are trained in many states!

Food allergy affects 3.7 % of all adults and an even higher number of children, with 6 to 8 % of children having food allergies. A food allergy is often characterized by symptoms described above, occurring within minutes to an hour of eating the offending food. Swelling of the mouth, throat, or tongue, a drop in blood pressure, nausea, dizziness, and/ or difficulty in breathing happen because the body produces proteins called antibodies that call out the troops to attack. Mostly this attack is a surge of histamine, and it can become life-threatening. This type of reaction is what we call *IgE-mediated*, and blood tests such as the ELISA (enzyme-linked immunosorbent assay) test will diagnose it. In addition, if you are diagnosed with one, you often carry an Epi-pen with you at all times in the event the food you are allergic to is in the meal you are eating.

FOOD INTOLERANCE

ELISA, a simple blood test, is sensitive and specific to the body's immune response. So sensitive that it can detect the presence of hormones, antibodies, and even the toxins secreted by bacteria. Though food allergy is a life and death matter and complete avoidance is the only preventive measure a person can take, another problem people suffer from is food *intolerance,* sometimes referred to as "delayed food intolerance," which involves a different set of proteins or immunoglobulins. With food intolerance, you may experience many of the same symptoms as those with food allergy but more commonly clients report stomach pain, joint inflammation, mood changes or headache. These symptoms can occur after eating the meal or begin the next day.

Two doctors who studied people with Chronic Fatigue Syndrome, Doctors Wong and Logan, found food intolerances cause many more things than digestive problems and fatigue. They can also cause joint inflammation, mood changes and pain.[45] Other researchers[46] using the ELISA test on Belgian people with this disease reported in 2006 their findings of elevated IgM responses to specific fats and proteins as a result of oxidative damage.

EXCUSE ME, YOUR GUT IS LEAKING!

When a food intolerance continues to happen without being identified and treated, you feel as though a freight train ran you over with nausea, headache, and aches from your stem to your sternum. In other words, flu symptoms develop as fever-producing chemicals called cytokines rush into the bloodstream, and you most likely become very depressed feeling this way every day. There is good news to this story; when the food intolerances are caught and treated by complete avoidance of the specific offenders, you get

---

[45] Logan, A.C., & Wong, C. (2001), Chronic fatigue syndrome : oxidative stress and dietary modifications. *Alternative Medicine Review* 6(5).
[46] Maes, M., Mihaylova, I., & Leunis, J.C. (2006) Chronic fatigue syndrome is accompanied by an IgM-related immune response directed against neopitopes formed by oxidative or nitrosative damage to lipids and proteins. *Neueroendocrinology Letters* 27(5).

your energy back and feel like singing and dancing to Pharrell's very popular song, "HAPPY!"

You might ask, why would my depression diminish from avoiding my favorite meatball hoagie with extra parmesan cheese? Because, sometimes the reaction to tomatoes or cheese causes emotional changes such as depression and anxiety. Individuals react to different foods. Not everyone reacts the same way to a given food. One of the activities going on in our intestines is the creation of our neurotransmitters. These are the chemicals our brain needs to function, such as norepinephrine, dopamine, and serotonin. We need the nutrients we take in to create these neurotransmitters. If we cannot process them because the cells in the intestine are damaged, think about how a disruption in this process of making the happy hormone, serotonin, can make a person feel!

Food intolerances arise from an intestinal wall allowing undigested food particles to leak out into the bloodstream, otherwise known as "leaky gut." The food particles are not supposed to be entering the bloodstream, so the intestinal wall is malfunctioning. The medical community is now starting to recognize this.[47] Early symptoms such as a drop in energy or difficulty concentrating may not first appear to involve the GI tract. The amount of food needed to trigger the symptoms is far greater than in food allergy. Remember, with a food allergy, just a drop of the offender could send the unlucky eater to the ER with a life-threatening swelling of the airways called *anaphylaxis*.

Food intolerance takes a while to develop. It might take months or years, and it's often our favorite food that betrays us. The first time I underwent testing for a delayed food allergy or food

---

[47] health.clevelandclinic.org/find-the-source-of-your-food-intolerance-and-finally-find-relief/ March 13, 2019

intolerance, I prayed that the test results measuring my IgG levels would return with zero antibodies to chocolate. I sure did not want to give up my drug of choice! I was lucky. However, my antibodies to fish, corn, and soy came back with the highest degree of reactivity, a +4.

So here we are: From the use of NSAIDS like ibuprofen and a low fiber diet and toxins, we now have porous cell membranes, with an intestinal liming damaged at the cellular level, poorly absorbing partially-digested food because our enzymes are not efficient at breaking food down and now food particles enter our bloodstream. The results are bloating, abdominal pain, fatigue, and low energy as the nutrients we need to build hormones, neurotransmitters, and create energy are not being utilized. We can add irritable and grouchy to the list. Do you know anyone who fits this description?

BACKED UP? CONGESTED?

I have counseled clients with a variety of symptoms from food intolerance. Some that are not GI symptoms at all: runny nose, headaches, a full feeling in the ears, difficulty concentrating, coughing, and subclinical constipation. What is that? It means not pooping in adequate amounts. Real *constipation*, the clinical term that doctors refer to, means only going three times a week - but our bodies need to have a daily elimination to stay healthy. Many of us with internal traffic jams go to the gastroenterologist to find out that nothing serious is wrong with us. After tests are done, the doctor hands us a sheet of paper with a list of high fiber foods and a recommendation to drink water. Other people reading this suffer from alternating constipation and diarrhea, fitting the description of IBS. You too, have seen the gastro- people who ran the full gamut of testing and ruling out pockets, cysts, and other abnormalities do not know what to do for you. So you end up living on antacids, laxatives, stool softeners, and pain killers. This is when seeing a nutritionist, preferably one who specializes in food allergies and intolerances, comes in handy. Nutritionists who specialize in feeding the body what it needs, may be able to help you find some relief. I also recommend Integrative medical doctors who understand how the brain hormones can affect the body in unusual ways and provide you with specific nutrients and amino acids that can correct imbalances.

With a food intolerance, it may take up to three consecutive days of eating corn in various forms, such as the popcorn you eat at the Sunday matinee, the corn tortilla you have on Monday, and the corn bread you eat with a hearty bowl of chili on Tuesday. Come Wednesday, you might feel very achy before leaving your bed. I have counseled people with intolerances to the proteins in another food, soy. With one client, no GI symptoms were ever experienced, but the client had constant sinus infections. His doctor put him on antibiotics for 14 days. He was free of infection for one or two weeks and then back on antibiotics again for another 14-day course. His body was reacting to the soy in his diet, and his ears were responding by accumulating fluid.

He would also lose his balance frequently and continued to suffer from painful ear infections until all the soy was removed from his diet. We had to hunt down every source of soy, including the soy protein isolate used as a filler in the frozen dinners he was eating every night. Once he stopped eating frozen dinners, and eliminated his favorite seasoning, soy sauce, his ear infections stopped, and the fluid that had been sitting around inside his ear canals was no longer present to provide a breeding ground for the bacteria that caused all of the infections.

With food intolerance, the immune system is constantly challenged by one or more specific foods such as milk for one person, wheat for another, creating antibodies to the perceived offender. It's as if the alarm system is constantly activated, so we live in a perpetually inflamed state. Our knowledge about the immune system is changing. Once believed to reside mainly in the spleen and lymph tissues, we now know that 80% of the immune system is right at the intestinal wall, where the food is absorbed into the blood. If you constantly eat something that the immune system incorrectly identifies as a foreign agent, your body works harder than it should, constantly on overdrive. Inside, you have more oxidative stress, more chemicals from the adrenal gland that controls blood sugar, flooding the bloodstream, and subsequently more work for those poor adrenal glands. In addition, the increased oxidative stress puts you at greater risk for heart disease and even cancer. The constant challenge to the intestines, integrative medical practitioners believe, can lead eventually to IBS and Crohn's disease.

SECTION 2

THE ENERGY PLAN

In the next few pages, I've created menus for 2 weeks. The daily nutrients you need are supplied in these menus, with no need to count calories. All the meals are what nutritionists refer to as "calorie-dense," meaning that the percentage of nutrients are greater than the calories, certainly nothing like the empty calories a devil's food cake provides. These are menus full of soluble fiber in the form of fruits and vegetables, and insoluble fiber from the whole grains. In addition, you will be using extra virgin olive oil for cooking and in your salad dressings. I am having you decrease consumption of the inflammatory omega 6 oils (corn, soybean, or anything hydrogenated). The omega 6 oils create inflammation compared to the omega 3 oils found in fish, which tamp down inflammation, and you can liberally use the neutral omega 9 oils found in nuts and olives) You may like the flavor of EVOO drizzled on fresh vegetables with a few herbs of your choice.

The meats and eggs you eat will be pasture-raised and organic so you receive top-notch omega-3 sources of protein that are free from antibiotics and hormones.

If you need to add salt to meals, please avoid table salt, which is created from two ingredients; sodium and chloride that directly raises blood pressure in some people. I recommend using a mineral salt that provides us sodium along with the trace minerals-selenium, manganese, and magnesium, which help drive the reactions in our body that create energy!

Instead of getting your energy from caffeinated sodas and continuous infusions of coffee, you will enjoy one cup of organic coffee at breakfast. And please put down the Red Bull or any energy-drinks containing guarana; It will only defeat the purpose. To help meet your calcium requirements, you will drink milk in the form that is best for you. Milk, you remember, contains PROTEIN and the energy-creating B-vitamins that you cannot get from a cup of coffee. For those who are lactose intolerant, you can add commercial lactase enzymes to organic whole milk. Alternatively, you can drink a calcium-enriched soy or almond based milk or turn to goat's milk. Check the carton's label to see that 33% or one-third of your calcium requirement is present in one serving comparable to cow's milk. (You may be wondering why you do not see rice milk in this list. Generally, rice milks only provide one gram of protein. There is one brand, Vitasoy Rice milk that supplies us with 7 grams of protein. You may use this if you have a soy and nut allergy.) I want you to gain the CLA from grass-fed whole milk when possible.

You will notice that there is no wine or beer or any alcohol in this program. This is not punishment. This is because:

1) Alcohol is an empty calorie food. It goes straight into the bloodstream from the intestinal wall and goes to the liver for processing. On its way, it can irritate the lining of the GI tract.

2) Every medicine we take, even something as simple as an aspirin, needs to be metabolized by the liver to be broken down. Anyone with a chronic illness has a liver that is already working very hard to process the medications we take.

3) We want to get rid of fuzzy brain syndrome, Covid-brain or Fibro-brain (it has a few cute names), and alcohol certainly contributes to muddled thinking. Alcohol also makes you frequently pee, further drying out the body and lowering the blood volume for those of you who contend with this issue.

This program is designed to make life EASIER so that you feel less harried and more relaxed around mealtimes. It's important to follow the meal plans as written and to not forget a meal. For snack foods that you will be bringing to work, such as bell pepper rings or goat's cheese, slice the food the night before and keep refrigerated. Ice water will keep the vegetables crisp.

Throughout the day, we need to drink plentiful amounts of water for many reasons; the water dilutes the saliva in our mouth, it moistens the food as we chew, and makes up a proportion of our blood volume. Water also is needed to complement fiber (roughage). Without adequate fluid, the fiber in some foods can become an immovable mass sitting in your intestines. You don't want this to happen. Did you know that water keeps our body temperature stable? You are most likely knowledgeable about the need to drink extra fluids in the warm weather months, but we need water year-round; and it is calorie-free so you can drink as much as 8 cups a day.

You will be starting the day with a rather large breakfast. It will certainly seem that way to you if you are currently eating an energy bar on the way out the door. Every morning you will drink either pomegranate or cranberry juice, high in antioxidants, and pomegranate contains *punicalagin*. This antioxidant improves the heart and lung function and protects the nervous system's cells from oxidative stress injury.[48] That is what this whole book is about: protecting your body from oxidative stress or ROS, which ages us and makes our cells old before their time. The meals contain whole grains and protein so that you will not become hungry an hour later the way you would if you had eaten a doughnut off the cart at work.

The snacks are necessary for you to obtain the calcium requirements from food, rather than supplements, and to consume the fiber everyone needs. The snacks are designed to keep you feeling satisfied with a blood sugar level that will stay on an even keel. In addition, you will find that they are all gluten-free snacks. As described in chapter 4, many of us with irritated intestines need to take a break from gluten-containing foods. Remember, our grandparents did not have extra gluten added to the bread they ate. Our intestines may not have adapted yet to the changed wheat flour that is found in breads, crackers, and cereals. Also, we don't yet know the effects of genetically modified foods on our bodies, so my theory is to avoid GMO's until the research on humans is completed. We don't want to be guinea pigs.

My focus as a nutritionist is to teach my clients how to eat well, not on taking supplements. However, I am frequently asked if there were one or two supplements that I would recommend; my recommendation is to take vitamin D3 and a multi-vitamin.

---

[48] Chen, B., Longtine M.S., & Nelson, D.M. Punicalagin, a polyphenol in pomegranate juice, downregulates p53 and attenuates hypoxia-induced apoptosis in cultured human placental syncytiotrophoblasts. *American Journal of Physiology-Endocrinology and Metabolism*, 305(10), E1274-E1280. ncbi.nim.nih.gov/pmc/articles/PMC3840214 Oct 1 2013.doi.10.1152/ajpendo.002188 2013

Vitamin D is a unique vitamin that our skin creates in the presence of sunshine. It is difficult to receive enough sunlight if you live in the upper latitude because the weather is not warm enough year-round to be without a coat or sweater. And in New England, the winter temperatures can be quite chilly and snowy, so we need scarves, hats, and gloves. The food sources of this vitamin are egg yolks, fish, and mushrooms. You would not want to eat these every day, so I do advise my clients to take a supplement of vitamin D3. This vitamin protects us against many cancers and is good for the immune system. I generally recommend the multi-vitamin to those with intestinal absorption problems since many of our vitamins are made in our intestines. When I first meet a client, I have him take one until I see the diet is more balanced.

One last very important bit of news: you will ditch your microwave oven for at least two weeks. I know they make life convenient, but the nutrient quality of foods is greatly diminished by microwaving foods. This is still controversial in traditional medical circles. Nevertheless, Spanish researchers compared the nutrients lost in microwaved broccoli (97%) to that of boiled (66%).[49] Also, studies done by researchers at the University of Damanhour at Egypt on mice given microwaved food for only eight weeks, showed an alteration in the biochemical pathways in the liver of mice. Specifically, the study found liver damage as well as a decrease in the crucial enzymes, *glutathione peroxidase*, and SOD, *superoxide dismutase*.[50] These enzymes actually destroy free

[49] Vallejo, F.A., Barberán, T., & Garicia-Viguera, C.J. Phenolic compound contents in edible part of broccoli inflorescences after domestic cooking *Journal of the Science of Food and Agriculture*. (2005) 83: 1511-1516.
[50] El Ghazaly, N. A., Kamel, K., Radwan, E.H., Said, H., & Barakat, A. (2014) Impact of microwave heated food on health.. *Journal of Advances in Biology* 5(3). academia.edu/8677956/impact_of_microwave_heated_food_on_health

radicals so having a lowered amount of them is dangerous to our health. Remember, our campaign is to prevent the accumulation of free radicals inside our bodies with the most anti-oxidant rich diet one can employ.

TO YOUR HEALTH!

2-WEEK MEAL PLAN

DAY 1

BREAKFAST

o   8 oz. of Pomegranate Juice, Mixed with 4 oz. of Water or Apple Juice
o   2 Gluten- free Waffles with Organic Vanilla Yogurt
o   Peaches or Mango Slices
o   1 Hardboiled Egg
o   Coffee or Green Tea

A.M. SNACK

o   1 Slice Gluten-free Bread with Melted Organic Cheddar Cheese

LUNCH

o   Shrimp Pad Thai Soup with Spinach **
o   1 Apple (or unsweetened apple sauce if unable to eat raw fruit)
o   Green Tea

AFTERNOON SNACK

o   Red Pepper Rings
o   Cucumber Slices
o   With up to 1/2 Cup of Yogurt with Dried Spices

DINNER

o   Perdue Organic Short Cuts Chicken Sprinkled with Pesto Sauce
o   French-style Green Beans
o   1 Sweet Potato
o   Herbal Tea

DESSERT

o   Pineapple Chunks or Slices Sprinkled with Coconut Flakes
o   8 oz. of Milk (of your choice)

DAY 2

BREAKFAST

o   8 oz. of Unsweetened Cranberry Juice
o   Instant Organic Oatmeal with Apricot Spread
o   2 Finn Crisp Rye Thins
o   8 oz. Milk (of your choice)
o   Coffee or Green Tea

A.M. SNACK

o   17 Blue Diamond Nut Crackers or 11 Good Thins GF crackers
o   1-2 oz. Soft Goat's Cheese, Herbed or Plain

LUNCH

o   1 Cup of Split Pea Soup
o   Yellowfin Tuna Salad with Scallions and Fresh Basil Leaf
o   Inside a Spelt or Gluten-free English Muffin**
o   10 Baby Carrots
o   One Banana
o   Hot or Iced Tea

AFTERNOON SNACK

o   Yasso Frozen Greek Yogurt Bar

DINNER

o   Organic Brown Rice Pasta with Marinara Sauce
o   1/2 Cup Mushrooms
o   Salad of 2 Cups Baby Greens, Grape Tomatoes

DESSERT

o   Cut Watermelon or 2 Date Almond or Coconut Rolls

DAY 3

BREAKFAST

o   4 oz. of Pomegranate Juice, Mixed with 4 oz. Water or Apple
    Juice
o   2 Slices of Gluten-free Bread, Toasted, with 2 Poached Eggs
o   Handful of Blueberries
o   Coffee or Green Tea

A.M. SNACK

o   2 Lundberg Rice Cakes Spread with Wholly Guacamole
o   2 Cherry Tomatoes
o   2 Slices Turkey Breast

LUNCH

o   1 Cup of Organic Butternut Squash Soup (Imagine or Pacific)
o   3 Deli Stuffed Grape Leaves
o   One Dr. Praeger's Heirloom Bean Veggie Burger
o   Dole Tropical Fruit Cup (in juice only)
o   Green Tea

AFTERNOON SNACK

o   8 oz of Organic Yogurt
o   Seasoned Rice Crackers

DINNER

o   ½ Gluten-free Spinach & Bell Pepper Pizza

DESSERT

o   1/2 Cup Blueberries or Crispy Blueberry Dessert
o   8 oz. Milk (of your choice)

DAY 4

BREAKFAST

o 4 oz. of Pomegranate Juice, Mixed with 4 oz. Water or Apple Juice

o Maddie's Choice Spelt or Gluten-free Bagel with Lox or Smoked Bluefish

o 2 slices of Organic Cheese

o 1 Apple

o Coffee or Green Tea

A.M. SNACK

o 8 oz. of Organic Peach Yogurt with 1/2 Cup Gluten-free Granola

LUNCH

o 1/2 carton of Imagine Mushroom Soup

o Gluten-free Crackers, (preferably without seeds)

o Fruit and Veggie Salad**

o Green Tea

AFTERNOON SNACK

o 10 Raw Bell Pepper Strips with Yogurt Dip

o 2 Finn Crisp Rye Thins

o 8 oz. of V8 Juice

DINNER

o Organic Ramen Noodles with Peas and Mushrooms

o 8 oz. of Milk (of your choice)

DESSERT

o Pineapple Chunks Scattered with coconut flakes

DAY 5

BREAKFAST

- o 4 oz. Pomegranate Juice, Mixed with 4 oz. Water or Apple Juice
- o Organic Corn Cereal with 1/2 Cup Fresh Strawberries
- o 1/2 Cup Milk
- o Two Corn Thins with Apricot Preserves
- o 1 Organic String Cheese
- o Coffee or Tea

A.M. SNACK

- o Against The Grain Gluten-free Pita Pocket Dipped in Artichoke Hummus

LUNCH

- o Organic Corn Pasta Medley with Pesto Sauce**
- o Bowl of European Mixed Greens with 1/2 Cup Chickpeas
- o Dole Tropical Fruit Cup in Juice & 4 Walnuts
- o Green Tea

AFTERNOON SNACK

- o Cucumber Slices with Maple Mustard Dressing*
- o Hard Boiled Egg

DINNER

- o 2 Organic Corn Tacos Filled with Ground Turkey, Red Kidney Beans
- o Green Leaf lettuce**
- o Peach Salsa and 1/2 Cup Muenster Cheese
- o Mixed Melon Cup
- o 8 oz of Milk (of your choice)

DESSERT

- o Banana "Ice Cream" Sundae*

DAY 6

BREAKFAST

o   4 oz. Pomegranate Juice
o   2 Gluten-free Waffles with 8 oz. of Organic Yogurt
o   1 Banana/tbsp. Crushed Walnuts
o   Coffee or Tea

A.M. SNACK

o   2 Tbsp. Almond Butter on Brown Rice Snaps by Edward & Sons
o   or 365 Day Brown Rice Crackers
o   8 oz. V8 juice

LUNCH

o   Organic Butternut Squash Soup
o   2 Cups Organic Baby Spinach Leaves
o   Prepared Black Bean & Corn Salad/or Chickpea or Lentil Salad
o   1 oz of Hard Cheese
o   Brown Rice Snaps
o   Red Grapes
o   Green Tea

AFTERNOON SNACK

o   Chocolate Milk

DINNER

o   Take-Out Thai Chicken with Peanuts
o   Broccoli or Spinach
o   1 Cup Brown Rice
o   Herbal Tea (of your choice)

DESSERT

o   Gluten-free Crackers Layered with Honey and Greek Yogurt

DAY 7

BREAKFAST
o 4 oz. Pomegranate Juice
o 2 Free-Range Eggs, Scrambled with 1/2 Cup Organic Cheese
o 2 Kamut Flatbreads
o 1-2 Maplegate Farms Chicken Sausage Patties
o 1/2 Cup Strawberries
o Coffee or Green Tea

A.M. SNACK
o Suzie's Sesame Kamut Flatbread
o 1.5 Ounces Goat's Cheese
o Crofter's Organic Just Fruit Spread Wild Blueberry

LUNCH
o Roast Pork Loin
o 1 Sweet Potato
o 1 Cup Unsweetened Applesauce
o Broccoli Salad from Deli
o 2 Slices Sprouted Grain Bread
o 8 oz. V8 Juice
o Green Tea

AFTERNOON SNACK
o Pear Slices with Vanilla Yogurt and 1/4 Cup Crushed Walnuts

DINNER
o 1 Cup Mushroom Soup
o Thai Chicken (leftover) & Baked Potato
o Salad of European Mixed Greens, Artichoke Hearts & Grated Carrot
o Amy's Organic Shiitake Vinaigrette Dressing

DESSERT
o Melon Cup

DAY 8

BREAKFAST
- o 4 oz Pomegranate Juice
- o 8 oz. of Organic Greek Yogurt
- o 4 oz. Gluten-free Granola Cereal with 1 Cup Blueberries
- o Coffee or Green Tea

A.M. SNACK
- o 2 Slices of Sprouted Grain Bread, Toasted
- o With up to 2 Tsp. Almond Butter

LUNCH
- o Organic Butternut Squash Soup
- o High Protein Salad** with Maple-mustard Dressing**
- o Green Tea

AFTERNOON SNACK
- o Red Pepper Hummus
- o 3 Finn Crisp Caraway Crispbread

DINNER
- o Amy's Organic Rice Macaroni and Cheese
- o Baby Spinach Salad with Chopped Walnuts
- o Mandarin Orange Slices and 1/2 Cup Fresh Raspberries

DESSERT
- o 1 Gluten-free Waffle with Mango or Peach Slices (and its juice)

DAY 9

BREAKFAST

- o 4 oz. Pomegranate Juice
- o 1 cup Organic Corn Cereal & One-half Cup Milk
- o 1/2 Cup Strawberries
- o 1 Hard Boiled Egg
- o Gluten-free Whole Grain Bread
- o Coffee or Green Tea

A.M. SNACK

- o V8 Juice
- o 2 Cups of Non-GMO Popcorn Dusted with Cheese

LUNCH

- o Roast Pork (left over from day 7) with Gravy
- o Served Open-faced on 2 Slices Gluten-free Whole Grain Bread
- o 1 Cup Frozen Organic Corn
- o Baby Spinach Salad*
- o 1 Pear
- o Green Tea

AFTERNOON SNACK

- o 8 oz. Organic Greek Yogurt & 4 oz. Gluten-free Granola Cereal

DINNER

- o 1 Cup of Organic New England Style Clam Chowder
- o Cedar's Mediterranean Lentil Salad on Bed of Boston Lettuce
- o 1 Cup of Quinoa Pilaf from the Deli
- o 1 oz of Gouda Cheese
- o 1 Bunch of Red Grapes

DESSERT

- o 1 cup Nature's Promise or SO Brand Coconut Non-dairy Dessert or Coconut Bliss (Luna & Larry's)
  Don't forget to cook millet in beef broth for tomorrow

DAY 10

BREAKFAST

o   8 oz. of Unsweetened Cranberry Juice
o   2 Poached Eggs on 2 Slices of Gluten-free Schär Bread, Toasted
o   1 Shelton Turkey Sausage Patty
o   Coffee or Green Tea

A.M. SNACK

o   3 Finn Crisp Caraway Rye Thins
o   1 oz. of Soft Goat's Cheese
o   1/2 Cup Blueberries

LUNCH

o   Yellowfin Tuna Salad
o   European Mixed Greens
o   8 Grape Tomatoes
o   1 Cup Mango Slices
o   Green Tea
o   2 Suzie's Rosemary Kamut Flatbread

AFTERNOON SNACK

o   Organic Greek Yogurt with 1 Cup Strawberries

DINNER

o   Organic, Free-range Hamburger in a Gluten-free Roll
o   Millet Mushroom Pilaf**
o   1 Cup Vegetarian Baked Beans
o   Deli Carrot Raisin Salad
o   2 Slices of Pineapple
o   8 oz of Milk

DESSERT

o   Cut Watermelon or 2 Date Almond Rolls or Coconut Rolls.

DAY 11

BREAKFAST

- o 4 oz. Pomegranate Juice
- o Maddie's Spelt Bagel
- o 1 Poached Egg with 1.5 Oz. of Organic Cheddar Cheese
- o Red Grapes
- o Coffee or Green Tea

A.M. SNACK

- o 1/4 cup Hummus
- o Raw or Lightly Steamed Baby Carrots and Broccoli Crowns

LUNCH

- o Tomato Soup with Shrimp, Mushrooms and Peas**
- o 2 Slices of Suzie's Seeded Spelt Flatbreads
- o 1/2 Cup of Mango
- o Green Tea

AFTERNOON SNACK

- o Greek Yogurt with Honey with 2 Dried Figs

DINNER

- o 4-5 ounces of Organic Free-range Beef
- o 1 Baked Sweet Potato
- o 1 Cup Baby Bok Choy Sautéed in EVOO
- o Un-caffeinated Beverage of Your Choice

DESSERT

- o 1/2 Cup of Pineapple Chunks with 1/2 Cup of Blueberries
- o Scattered Coconut Flakes

DAY 12

BREAKFAST

o   4 oz. of Pomegranate Juice
o   Hot Quinoa Flakes Cereal
o   2 Tbsp. of Almond Butter
o   1 Cup Mandarin Orange Slices
o   Coffee or Green Tea

A.M. SNACK

o   8 oz of Organic Greek Yogurt
o   1 Pear Sprinkled with Cinnamon
o   1 Organic Popcorn Cake

LUNCH

o   One Cup of Amy's Black Bean Soup
o   2 Small Soft Corn Tortillas Filled with Cheese and Tomato
o   Artichoke Hearts
o   1 Cup Strawberries
o   Green Tea

AFTERNOON SNACK

o   Hot Cocoa and 2 Cups of Non-GMO Popcorn

DINNER

o   Lentil Soup or Kettle Cuisine Thai Curry Chicken Soup
o   Stuffed Grape Leaves from the Deli Section
o   Carrot Raisin Salad

DESSERT/SNACK

o   3 Cups of Non-GMO Popcorn

DAY 13

BREAKFAST

o 4 oz. Pomegranate Juice
o Instant Organic Oatmeal with ¼ Cup Sliced Almonds
o 1 Hard Boiled Egg
o Coffee or Green Tea

A.M. SNACK

o 1-2 oz. Soft Goat's Cheese on Finn Crisp Rye Thins
o 1 Pear

LUNCH

o 2 Slices of Oatmeal Bread
o 4 oz of Crabmeat
o Rosemary Mayonnaise**
o Green Leaf Lettuce
o Red Grapes and Walnuts
o Green Tea

AFTERNOON SNACK

o Organic Yogurt
o GF Crackers and 2 Slices Dried or Fresh Mango

DINNER

o 1 Salmon Patty (wild ocean caught)
o 1 Cup of Brown Rice with ½ Cup of Raisins
o Cooked Carrots
o Prepared Broccoli Salad from Deli
o 8 oz. Milk (of your choice)

DESSERT

o Date Banana Rolls

DAY 14

BREAKFAST

- o 4 oz of Pomegranate Juice
- o 1 Poached Egg on Gluten-free English Muffin, Toasted
- o 1 Slice of Organic Cheddar Cheese
- o 1/2 Cup Blueberries
- o Coffee or Tea

A.M. SNACK

- o 8 Brown Rice Snaps
- o 2 Tbsp. Almond Butter
- o 1 Apple

LUNCH

- o Hearty Black Bean Soup
- o European Greens Salad
- o Grape Tomatoes & Organic Dressing of Your Choice
- o 6-8 Gluten-free Crackers without Seeds

AFTERNOON SNACK

- o 4 oz. Greek Yogurt with 1/2 Cup Apples and Cinnamon
- o 1/4 Cup Gluten-free Granola

DINNER

- o BBQ Rotisserie Chicken (pre-cooked)
- o Organic Baby Spinach, Cooked
- o Baked Sweet Potato
- o Pineapple Slices
- o 1-2 Slices of Sprouted Grain Bread

DESSERT

- o 1 Cup Luna & Larry's Chocolate Coconut Bliss Non-dairy Dessert

RECIPES

SHRIMP PAD THAI SOUP WITH SPINACH

INGREDIENTS

- o 10 shrimp, cooked and cleaned
- o 1 cup of Dr. McDougall's Pad Thai
- o 1 large handful of baby spinach

PREPARATION

1. Defrost the shrimp 1 hour ahead of time in a bowl of cool water. Discard the water.
2. Remove the tails from the shrimp.
3. Open the Pad Thai and pour boiled water into the Pad Thai up to the line in the cup. Allow it to stand for required time on the package.
4. Into a clean saucepan, add the pad Thai.
5. Stir in the spinach and shrimp.

BANANA "ICE CREAM" SUNDAE

INGREDIENTS

- o 1 banana
- o 1 scoop non-dairy dessert (coconut based) I recommend: Stop & Shop's Nature's Promise Free from Chocolate Coconut non-dairy dessert; SO Delicious Brand Chocolate Coconut non-dairy dessert; or Luna & Larry's Dark Chocolate Coconut Bliss.
- o toasted coconut flakes

PREPARATION

1. Peel the banana and split lengthwise.
2. Add a scoop of non-dairy dessert and garnish with Toasted coconut flakes.

QUICK BLUEBERRY CRUMBLE

INGREDIENTS

- o   1 cup fresh blueberries
- o   1 pkg. instant organic oatmeal (apple flavor)
- o   1 tbsp. coconut oil
- o   Pure Maple Syrup
- o   one small (approx. 6 x 7) baking pan

PREPARATION

1. Set oven to 350°F.
2. Rinse blueberries then place in pan
3. Open the package of oatmeal and sprinkle it over the berries.
4. Melt 1 tbsp. coconut oil on low heat and then drizzle it over the mix.
5. Use a thin trickle of maple syrup on top of this and place in oven.
6. Bake for 12 minutes

ROSEMARY MAYONNAISE

INGREDIENTS

- o   1/8 Tsp. dried Rosemary
- o   1/4 cup Miracle Whip Dressing or mayonnaise of your choice
- o   1/8 Tsp. garlic powder

PREPARATION

1. Crumble the Rosemary in your hands. It needs to be broken up. Combine the ingredients with a wire Whisk.

Makes 2 servings

MAPLE MUSTARD DRESSING

INGREDIENTS

- o 1 tbsp. Extra Virgin Olive Oil
- o 1 tsp. maple syrup
- o 1 tsp. prepared yellow or grain mustard, such as Grey Poupon

PREPARATION

1. Combine all ingredients using a wire whisk and beat until smooth.

HIGH PROTEIN SALAD

INGREDIENTS

- o 6 romaine lettuce leaves
- o 1/2 cup canned chickpeas
- o 1 hard-boiled egg, sliced
- o 1/2 cup grated carrot
- o 10 grape tomatoes
- o 1/2 sliced cucumber
- o 8 black olives
- o ½ cup of organic shredded cheese

PREPARATION

1. To a bed of lettuce leaves, arrange the vegetables any way you like. Serve with maple-mustard dressing.

YELLOW FIN TUNA SALAD

INGREDIENTS

- o 1 can of yellow fin tuna
- o 2 tablespoons of commercial mayonnaise
- o 1 scallion, sliced
- o fresh basil leaf
- o 2 leaves of Boston Bibb lettuce

PREPARATION

1. Combine the tuna with the mayonnaise and one scallion.
2. Add one half leaf of fresh basil, cut with scissors.
3. Place on a bed of Boston lettuce.

Makes 2 Servings

BANANA COCONUT "SUNDAE"

INGREDIENTS

- o 1 banana sliced lengthwise
- o 1 scoop of Luna and Larry's Naked Coconut Bliss
- o 1 tbsp of sliced almonds

PREPARATION

1. Place two halves of banana on a plate.
2. To this add the Coconut Bliss on top then sprinkle the nuts, Enjoy.

CORN PASTA MEDLEY

INGREDIENTS

- o 1 cup of mixed frozen vegetables (e.g. Italian Mix))
- o 1 pkg. corn pasta shells
- o 1 pkg. of dry pesto sauce
- o 1 Tbsp. EVOO
- o 1/2 tsp. water

PREPARATION

1. Cook pasta according to package directions.
2. During the last 5 min of cooking time, add the frozen vegetables to the water.
3. While this heats, mix 1 Tbsp. Pesto with oil and the water
4. Mix thoroughly with wire whisk.
5. Drain the pasta and vegetables in a colander.
6. Return to pan and toss the pasta with the pesto sauce. Serve.

FRUIT AND VEGGIE SALAD

INGREDIENTS

- o 2 cups mixed greens
- o 1 can of mandarin orange segments
- o 5 sliced shiitake mushrooms
- o strips of Swiss cheese to equal 2 ounces (depending on how it is sliced)
- o Annie's organic light Poppyseed dressing

PREPARATION

1. Arrange the greens on the plate.
2. Add the other ingredients and drizzle with the dressing.

APPLE CHEDDAR MELT

INGREDIENTS

- 1-2 slices of brown rice bread, or gluten free bread, defrosted
- 1 oz. organic cheddar cheese
- 1 apple, sliced
- ground cinnamon

PREPARATION

1. Place bread topped with cheese underneath the broiler (toaster oven is fine). Broil at least 1 inch away from the top of the broiler until the cheese melts and bubbles.
2. Top with apples slices and sprinkle with cinnamon.

SPINACH PIZZA

INGREDIENTS

- 1 frozen GF or cauliflower pizza
- 1 cup baby spinach
- 1/2 cup sliced yellow pepper
- chopped dried onion

PREPARATION

1. Follow package directions to preheat oven.
2. Arrange with baby spinach, bell pepper and onion.
3. Bake for 15 min or as the package of the crust recommends. Remove from oven.
4. Drizzle with Extra Virgin Olive before serving.

SNOW-CAPPED PINEAPPLES

INGREDIENTS

- o 1 cup of pineapple chunks
- o 1 tbsp. un-sulfured coconut flakes

PREPARATION

1. Open the can of pineapple chunks.
2. Pour contents into a small bowl.
3. Sprinkle with coconut flakes.

MUSHROOM MILLET PILAF

INGREDIENTS

- o 1 1/3 cups beef broth
- o 1/4 cup dry millet
- o 1 scallion, snipped with scissors
- o 1 can sliced mushroom
- o sprinkle dried Thyme
- o ground black pepper

PREPARATION

1. Heat the millet in the beef broth with the thyme, and scallions until the grain is fully absorbed. (This can be done ahead of time).
2. Then add mushrooms.
3. Sprinkle with freshly ground black pepper.

FRUIT 'N NUTS

INGREDIENTS

- o 1 container of tropical fruit
- o 1 tbsp. chopped walnuts

PREPARATION

1. Sprinkle the walnuts on top of the tropical fruit.

TURKEY TACOS

INGREDIENTS

- o 2 organic taco shells, such as Garden of Eatin' brand
- o 16 oz ground turkey
- o 1 pkg. of organic taco seasoning
- o 1/2 can of cooked red kidney beans
- o green leaf lettuce
- o peach salsa
- o 1 1/2 ounces shredded Muenster cheese

PREPARATION

1. Heat the meat in enough water to cover the pan over medium heat.
2. Stir the meat with a wooden spoon to break it up.
3. Cook until it is no longer pink.
4. Add the seasoning packet and enough water to total 1 cup. Stir well.
5. Rinse the beans under cool running water add to the meat.
6. Heat the tacos in oven if desired
7. Line each tortilla with green leaf lettuce.
8. Layer with turkey, cooked beans, and cheese.
9. Add a dollop of peach salsa to each.

TOMATO SOUP WITH MUSHROOMS & PEAS

INGREDIENTS

- o 1 can of your favorite tomato soup
- o 1 cup frozen peas
- o 1 small can of mushrooms, drained
- o 1 cup of cooked brown rice

PREPARATION

1. Prepare the soup according to the directions listed on the label.
2. Once it is mixed well, add the mushrooms and peas. Stir over medium heat.
3. Stir in one cup of cooked brown rice just before you serve.

BABY SPINACH SALAD

INGREDIENTS

- o 2 cups baby spinach
- o 1/2 cup raspberries
- o 1 can of mandarin orange segments
- o 1/4 cup walnut pieces

PREPARATION

1. Create a bed with the baby spinach.
2. Place the other ingredients on top.
3. Serve with your favorite organic dressing.

INDEX

A

B

C

D

E

F

G

H

I

K

Q

R

S

W

Y

Z

REFERENCES BY CHAPTER

Chapter 2 Frozen, Take-out and Ready to Eat

[1] Rennard, B.O., Ertl, R.F., Gossman, G.L., Robbins, R.A., & Rennard, S.I. (2000). Chicken soup inhibits neutrophil chemotaxis in vitro. *Chest*, 118(4), 1150-1157. https://doi.org/10.1378/chest.118.4.1150

[2] Babizhayev, M.A., Deyev, AI, and Yegorov, Y.E. Non-hydrolyzed in digestive tract and blood natural L-carnosine peptide ("bioactivated Jewish Penicillin") as a panacea of tomorrow for various flu ailments: signaling activity attenuating nitric oxide (NO) production, cytostasis, and NO-dependent inhibitor of influenza virus replication in macrophage in the human body infected with the virulent swine influenza A (H1N1) virus. *Journal of Basic and Clinical Physiology and Pharmacology*, 24(1), 1-26.

[3] Melzer, D., Rice, N.E., Lewis, C., Henley, W.E., & Galloway, T.S. (2010). Association of urinary bisphenol- a concentration with heart disease: evidence from NHANES 2003/06. *PLOS one*, 5(1), e8673

[4] Culkin, K.A ., & Fung, Y,C. Destruction of E. Coli and Salmonella typhimurium in Microwave-cooked soups *Journal of Milk Food Technology*. Vol 38, No. 1 Pages 8-15, January 1975

[5] Fung, D.Y.C., & Cunningham, F.E. (1980) 43(8): 641-650 Effect of Microwaves on Microorganisms in Foods. *Journal of Food Protection.* https://doi.org/10.4315/0362-028X-43.8.641

[6] Bates, C.J. & and Spencer, R.C. Survival of Salmonella species in eggs poached using a microwave oven. *Journal of Hospital Infection, 29(2), 121-127.* https://doi.org/10.1016/0195-6701(95)90193-0

[7] http://www.lessemf.com/mw-stnds.html microwave oven radiation hazards & standards. US Food and Drug Administration, HHS1030.10

Chapter 3 More Unprocessed Grains

[8] Nasiadek, M., Stragierowicz, J., Klimczak, M., & Kilanowicz, A. The role of zinc in selected female reproductive system disorders. *Nutrients*, (2020)12(8), 2464 https://doi.org/10.3390/nu12082464

[9] Fung, T.T., Hu, F.B., Pereira, M.A., Liu, S., Stampfer, M.J., Colditz, G.A., & Willett, W.C. (2002) Whole-grain intake and the risk of type 2 diabetes: a prospective study in men. *The American journal of clinical nutrition*, 76(3), 535-540.

[10] Zunli, K., Yu, P., Xiodan, X. Chao, N., and Zhou, Z. *Citrus* flavonoids and Human Cancers. *Journal of Food and Nutrition Research.* (2015) 201 3(5): 341-357. https://doi.org/10.12691/JFNR-3-5-9

[11] Jaganathan, S.K., Vellayappan, M.V., Narasimhan, G., & Supriyanto, E. Role of pomegranate and citrus fruit juices in colon cancer prevention. *World Journal of Gastroenterology* (2014) Apr 28; 20(16): 4618-4625. https://doi.org/10.3748/wjg.v20.46.4618

[12] McKeown, N.M., Meigs, J.B., Liu, S., Wilson, P.W., & Jacques, P.F. (2002). Whole-grain intake is favorably associated with metabolic risk factors for type 2 diabetes and cardiovascular diseases in the Framingham Offspring Study. *American Journal of clinical nutrition,* 76(2).390-398. https://doi.org/10/1093/ajcn/762.390

Chapter 4 Snacks

[13] St.- Onge, M.P., Ard, J., Buskin, M.L., Chiuve, S.E., Johnson H.M., Etherton, P.K., and Varady, K. Meal Timing and Frequency: Implications for Cardiovascular Disease Prevention: A Scientific Statement from the American Heart Association. *Circulation* https://doi.org/10.1161/CIR0000000000000476/circulation.2017;135:e96-e121

Chapter 5 Interchangeable Meals

[14] Kennedy, A., Martinez, K., Schmidt, S., Mandrup, S., LaPoint, K., & McIntosh, M. Anti-obesity mechanisms of actions of conjugated linoleic acid. *The Journal of Nutritional Biochemistry,* 21(3), 171-179 https://doi.org/10.1016/j.jnutbio.2009.08.003

[15] Fulle, S., Mecocci, P., Fano, G., Vecchiet, I. Vecchini, A., Racciotti, D., & Beal. M.F. (2000) Specific Alterations in vastus lateralis muscle of patients with the diagnosis of chronic fatigue syndrome. *Free Radical Biology and Medicine,* 29(12), 1252-1259.

[16] Verma, C., Nanda, K., Singh, S. K., Singh, R. B.,. & Mishra, S. (2011) A review on impacts of genetically modified food on human health. *The Open Neutraceuticals Journal*, 4(1)3-11
https://www.doi.org/10.2174/1876396000110401

[17] Pitchford, Paul, (2002). *Healing with whole foods*: Asian traditions and modern nutrition. North Atlantic Books.

Chapter 6 From the Refrigerated Case

[18] Roberts, J. E. & Dennison, J. (2015). The Photobiology of lutein and zeaxanthin in the eye. *Journal of Ophthalmology*. (2015); Dec 20
https://www.doi.org/10.1155/2015/687173

[19] Fernandez, M.L. (2006). Dietary cholesterol provided by eggs and plasma lipoproteins in healthy populations. *Current Opinion in Clinical Nutrition & Metabolic Care*. 9(1), 8-12

[20] Vander Wal, J.S., Gupta, A., Khosla, P., & Dhurandhar, N.V. (2008) Egg breakfast enhances weight loss. *International Journal of Obesity*, 32(10), 1545-1551

[21] Benjamin S., & Spener, F. (2009). Conjugated linoleic acids as functional food: an insight into their health benefits. *Nutrition & Metabolism*, 6(1), 36.

Chapter 7 Fighter Nutrients from Fruits and Vegetables

[22] Grimm, K.A., Blanck, H.M., Scanlon, K.S., Moore, L.V., Grummer-Strawn, L.M., & Foltz, J.L. (2010). State-specific trends in fruit and vegetable consumption among adults-United States, 2000-2009. *Morbidity and Mortality Weekly Report*, 59(35), 1125-1130

[23] CDC Press Releases (2016, January 1). Retrieved from
http://www.cdc.gov/media/releases/2017/p1116-fruit-vegetable-consumption-html

[24] Papas, M.A., Giovannucci, E., & Platz, E.A. (2004). Fiber from fruit and colorectal neoplasia. *Cancer Epidemiology and Prevention Biomarkers,* 13(8), 1267-1270. http://cebp.aactjournalis.org/content/13/8/1267

[25] Racciatti, D., Vecchiet, J., Ceccomancini, A., Ricci, F., & Pizzigallo, E. (2001). Chronic fatigue syndrome following a toxic exposure. *Science of the total environment,* 270(1-3), 27-31.

[26] Rana, S., & Bhushan, S. (2016). Apple phenolics as nutraceuticals: assessment, analysis and application. *Journal of food science and technology,* 53(4), 1727-1738.

[27] Gao, Q., Qin, L. Q., Arafa, A., Eshak, E.S.,& Dong, J.Y. (2020) Effects of strawberry intervention on cardiovascular risk factors: A meta-analysis of randomised controlled trials. *British Journal of. Nutrition*; 124(3): 241-246. doi:10.1017/S000711452000121X

[28] Calvano, A., Izuora, K., Oh, E.C.,Ebersole, J.L., Lyons, T.J., & Basu, A. (2019). Dietary berries, insulin resistance, and type 2 diabetes: an overview of human feeding trials. *Food & Function* 10(10, 6227-6243 doi.10.1039/c9fo01426h

[29] Kolonel, L.N., Hankin, J.H., Whittemore, A.S., Wu, A.H., Gallagher, R.P., Wilkens, L.R. & Paffenbarger, R.S. (2000). Vegetables, fruits, legumes and prostate cancer: a multiethnic case-control study. *Cancer Epidemiology and Prevention Biomarkers,* 9(8), 795-804.

[30] Murray, C.W., Egan, S.K., Kim, H., Beru, N., & Bolger, P.M. (2008). U.S. Food and drug administration's total diet study: Dietary intake of perchlorate and iodine. *Journal of Exposure science and Environmental Epidemiology 18, 571-580*

[31] Melton III, L. J., (2003). Adverse outcomes of osteoporotic fractures in the general population. *Journal of Bone and Mineral Research,* 18(6), 1139-1141. https://doi.org/10.1359/jbmr.2003.18.6.1139

[32] Office of Dietary Supplements -Vitamin D. (n.d.) Retrieved from https://ods.od/nih.gov/factsheets/Vitamin D--Health Professional/

Chapter 8 The Geography of Food

[33] World Research Cancer Fund UK. (n.d.) *International* http://www.wcrf.org/

Chapter 9 The Beverage Cart

[34] Philion, C., Ma, D., Ruvinov, I., Mansour, F., Pignanelli, C., Noel, M. & Pandy, S. (2017) Cymbopogon citratus and Camellia sinensis extracts selectively induce apoptosis in cancer cells and reduce growth of lymphoma xenografts in vivo. *Oncotarget, 8(67), 110756*

[35] Xu, R., Yang, K., Ding, J., & Chen, G. (2010). Effect of green tea supplementation on blood pressure: A systematic review and meta-analysis of randomized controlled trials. *Medicine* Feb 2020 Vol 99 (6) doi:10.1097/MD.0000000000019047

[36] Wu, C.H., Yao, W.J., Lu, F.H., Wu, J.S., & Chang, C.J. (2002). Epidemiological Evidence of Increased Bone Mineral Density in Habitual Tea Drinkers. *Archives of internal Medicine*,162(9), 1001-1006 http://doi:10.1001/archinte.162.9.1001

[37] Swithers, S.E. (2013). Artificial sweeteners produce the counterintuitive effect of inducing metabolic derangements. *Trends in Endocrinology & Metabolism*, 24(9), 431-441 https://doi.org.10.1016/j.tem.2013.05.005

[38] Nettleton, J.A., Lutsey, P.L., Wang, Y., Lima, J.A., Michos, E.D., & Jacobs, D.R. (2009). Diet Soda intake and risk of Incident metabolic syndrome and type 2 diabetes in the multi-ethnic study of atherosclerosis (MESA). *Diabetes Care*, 32(4) 688-694 http://doi.org/10.2337/dc08-1799

[39] Li, X., Liu, Y., Wang, Y., Liu, X., Guo, M.,...& Jiang, M. (2020). Sucralose promotes colitis-associated colorectal cancer risk in a murine model along with changes in microbiota. *Frontiers in Oncology*, 10, 710 http://doi/10.3389/fonc.2020.00710

[40] Qin, X. (2012). Etiology of inflammatory bowel disease: a unified hypothesis. *World Journal of Gastroenterology* WJG,18(15), 1708 doi: 10.3748/wjg.v18.i15.1708

[41] de Koning, L., Malik, V.S., Kellogg, M.D., Rimm, E.B., Willett, W.C., & Hu, F.B. (2018) Sweetened beverage consumption, incident coronary heart disease, and biomarkers of risk in men. *Circulation* 125(14), 1735-1741. doi.org/10.1161/CIRCULATIONAHA.111.067017

[42] Yu, Z., Ley, S.H.,Sun, Q., Hu, F.B., & Malik, V.S. (2018). Cross-sectional association between sugar-sweetened beverage intake and cardiometabolic biomarkers in U.S. women. *British Journal of Nutrition*, 119(5), 570-580. DOI:
https://doi.org/10.1017/s0007114517000384

[43] Sonestedt, E., Øverby, N., Laaksonen, D., & Eva Birgisdottir, B. (2012). Does high sugar consumption exacerbate cardiometabolic risk factors and increase the risk of type 2 diabetes and cardiovascular disease? *Food and Nutrition Research*, 56(1), 19104.
ncbi.nim.nih.gov/pmc/articles/PMC3409338/doi:10.3402/fnr.v56i0.19104

[44] Duarte, S., Gregoire, S., Singh, A.P., Vorsa, N., Schaich, K., Bowen, W.H., & Koo, H. Inhibitory effects of cranberry polyphenols on formation of streptococcus mutans biofilms. *FEMS Microbiology Letters*, (2006) 257(1), 50-56. http://doi.org/10.1111/j.1574-6968.2006.00147

CHAPTER 11 Food Allergies and Intolerances

[45] Logan, A.C., & Wong, C. (2001) Chronic fatigue syndrome: oxidative stress and dietary modifications. Alternative Medicine Review, 6(5).

[46] Maes, M., Mihaylova, I. & Leunis, J.C., Chronic fatigue syndrome is accompanied by an IgM-related immune response directed against neopitopes formed by oxidative or nitrosative damage to lipids and proteins. *Neuroendocrinology Letters* 27(5):615-621

[47] health.clevelandclinic.org/find-the-source-of-your-food- intolerance-and-finally-find-relief. March 13, 2019.

PART II

[48] Chen, B., Longtine M.S., & Nelson, D.M. Punicalagin, a polyphenol in pomegranate juice, downregulates p53 and attenuates hypoxia-induced apoptosis in cultured human placental syncytiotrophoblasts. *American Journal of Physiology-Endocrinology and Metabolism*, 305(10), E1274-E1280.
ncbi.nim.nih.gov/pmc/articles/PMC384021.doi.10.1152/alpendo.002188 2013.

[49] Vallejo, F., Tomás-Barberán, F.A., & Garcia-Viguera, C. (2003) Phenolic compound contents in edible parts of broccoli inflorescences after domestic cooking *Journal of the Science of Food and Agriculture*, 83(14), 1511-1516.

[50] El Ghazaly, N.A., Kamel, K., Radwan, E.H., Said, H. & Barakat, A. (2014) Impact of microwave heated food on health. *Journal of Advances in Biology* 5 (3).
academia.edu/8677967/impact_of_microwave_heated_food_on_health

ABOUT THE AUTHOR

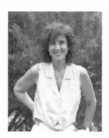

Mary L. Higgins, B.S., M.Ed. is a woman with fatiguing illness who shares the simple eating plan that made her feel better. She understands how important health-full eating is to a life filled with vitality and improved mood. Mary is a nutritionist who blogged for the NOURISH food blog with the Peabody Institute Library and a columnist for North Shore Children and Families Magazine. She teaches people how to live better through good nutrition.